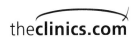

theclinics.com

CLINICS IN PERINATOLOGY

Medical Legal Issues in Perinatal Medicine: Part I

GUEST EDITORS
Isaac Blickstein, MD
Judith L. Chervenak, MD, JD
Frank A. Chervenak, MD

June 2007 • Volume 34 • Number 2

An Imprint of Elsevier, Inc.
PHILADELPHIA   LONDON   TORONTO   MONTREAL   SYDNEY   TOKYO

W.B. SAUNDERS COMPANY
A Division of Elsevier Inc.

Elsevier, Inc., 1600 John F. Kennedy Blvd., Suite 1800, Philadelphia, PA 19103-2899

http://www.theclinics.com

CLINICS IN PERINATOLOGY
June 2007
Editor: Carla Holloway

Volume 34, Number 2
ISSN 0095-5108
ISBN-10: 1-4160-4292-X
ISBN-13: 978-1-4160-4292-1

Reprints. For copies of 100 or more of articles in this publication, please contact the commercial Reprints Department, Elsevier Inc., 360 Park Avenue South, New York, New York 10010-1710. Tel: (212) 633-3813 Fax: (212) 462-1935, e-mail: reprints@elsevier.com.

The ideas and opinions expressed in *Clinics in Perinatology* do not necessarily reflect those of the Publisher. The Publisher does not assume any responsibility for any injury and/or damage to persons or property arising out of or related to any use of the material contained in this periodical. The reader is advised to check the appropriate medical literature and the product information currently provided by the manufacturer of each drug to be administered, to verify the dosage, the method and duration of administration or contraindications. It is the responsibility of the treating physician or other health care professional, relying on independent experience and knowledge of the patient, to determine drug dosages and the best treatment for the patient. Mention of any product in this issue should not be construed as endorsement by the contributors, editors, or the Publisher of the product or manufacturers' claims.

Clinics in Perinatology (ISSN 0095-5108) is published in quarterly by Elsevier Inc., 360 Park Avenue South, New York, NY 10010-1710. Months of issue are March, June, September, and December. Business and Editorial offices: 1600 John F. Kennedy Blvd., Suite 1800, Philadelphia, PA 19103-2899. Customer Service Office: 6277 Sea Harbor Drive, Orlando, FL 32887-4800. Periodicals postage paid at New York, NY and additional mailing offices. Subscription prices are $182.00 per year for (US individuals), $270.00 per year for (US institutions), $215.00 per year (Canadian individuals), $335.00 per year (Canadian institutions), $248.00 per year (foreign individuals), $335.00 per year (foreign institutions) $88.00 per year (US students), and $121.00 per year (foreign students). Foreign air speed delivery is included in all Clinics subscription prices. All prices are subject to change without notice. **POSTMASTER:** Send address changes to *Clinics in Perinatology*; Elsevier Periodicals Customer Service, 6277 Sea Harbor Drive, Orlando, FL 32887-4800. **Customer Service: 1-800-654-2452 (US). From outside of the US, call 1-407-345-1000.** E-mail: elspcs@elsevier.com

Clinics in Perinatology is also pubilshed in Spanish by McGraw-Hill Interamericana Editores S.A., P.O. Box 5-237, 06500 Mexico D.F., Mexico.

Clinics in Perinatology is covered in *Index Medicus, Current Contents, Excepta Medica, BIOSIS* and *ISI/BIOMED.*

Printed in the United States of America.

GUEST EDITORS

ISAAC BLICKSTEIN, MD, Department of Obstetrics and Gynecology, Kaplan Medical Center, Rehovot; and the Hadassah-Hebrew University School of Medicine, Jerusalem, Israel

JUDITH L. CHERVENAK, MD, JD, Clinical Assistant Professor of Obstetrics and Gynecology, New York University School of Medicine; of Counsel, Heidell, Pittoni, Murphy & Bach, LLP; Clinical Assistant, Professor of Obstetrics and Gynecology, New York University School of Medicine, New York, New York

FRANK A. CHERVENAK, MD, Given Foundation Professor and Chairman; Obstetrician; Gynecologist-in-Chief, Department of Obstetrics and Gynecology, Joan and Sanford I. Weill Medical College of Cornell University, The New York Presbyterian Hospital, New York, New York

CONTRIBUTORS

ISAAC BLICKSTEIN, MD, Department of Obstetrics and Gynecology, Kaplan Medical Center, Rehovot; and the Hadassah-Hebrew University School of Medicine, Jerusalem, Israel

ROBERT L. BRENT, MD, PhD, DSC (HON), Distinguished Professor of Pediatrics, Pathology, and Radiology; Louis and Bess Stein Professor of Pediatrics, Laboratory of Clinical and Environmental Teratology, Alfred I. DuPont Hospital for Children, Wilmington, Delaware

FRANK A. CHERVENAK, MD, Given Foundation Professor and Chairman; Obstetrician; Gynecologist-in-Chief, Department of Obstetrics and Gynecology, Joan and Sanford I. Weill Medical College of Cornell University, The New York Presbyterian Hospital, New York, New York

JUDITH L. CHERVENAK, MD, JD, Clinical Assistant Professor of Obstetrics and Gynecology, New York University School of Medicine; of Counsel, Heidell, Pittoni, Murphy & Bach, LLP; and Clinical Assistant, Professor of Obstetrics and Gynecology, New York University School of Medicine, New York, New York

WAYNE R. COHEN, MD, Chairman of Obstetrics and Gynecology, Jamaica Hospital Medical Center, Jamaica; Professor, Clinical Obstetrics and Gynecology, Department of Obstetrics and Gynecology, Weill Medical College of Cornell University, New York, New York

WILLIAM M. HUANG, MD, Maternal Fetal Medicine Fellow, Division of Maternal Fetal Medicine, Department of Obstetrics and Gynecology, New York University Medical Center, New York, New York

ROGER D. KLEIN, MD, JD, Research Affiliate, Department of Genetics, Yale University School of Medicine, New Haven, Connecticut

MAURICE J. MAHONEY, MD, JD, Professor of Genetics, Pediatrics, and Obstetrics, Gynecology & Reproductive Sciences, Department of Genetics, Yale University School of Medicine, New Haven, Connecticut

LAURENCE B. MCCULLOUGH, PhD, Professor of Medicine and Medical Ethics, Center for Medical Ethics and Health Policy, Baylor College of Medicine, Houston, Texas

ROBERT ROTH, BA, LLB, Sommers & Roth, Professional Corporation, Toronto, Ontario, Canada

BARRY S. SCHIFRIN, MD, Consulting Obstetrician, Department of Obstetrics and Gynecology, Kaiser Permanente—Los Angeles Medical Center, Los Angeles, California

DAVID E. SEUBERT, MD, JD, Assistant Professor of Obstetrics and Gynecology; Director, Medical Student Clerkship; Director of Obstetrics-Bellevue Hospital; Co-Director of Regional Perinatal Center-Bellevue Hospital, Division of Maternal Fetal Medicine, Department of Obstetrics and Gynecology, New York University Medical Center, New York, New York

RANDI WASSERMAN-HOFF, MD, Assistant Professor of Clinical Pediatrics; Co-Director of Regional Perinatal Center-Bellevue Hospital, Division of Neonatology, Department of Pediatrics, New York University Medical Center, New York, New York

CONTENTS

Overview of Professional Liability   227

Judith L. Chervenak

> Eighty-nine percent of American College of Obstetricians and
> Gynecologists fellows responding to the 2006 Professional Liability
> Survey indicated that they had been sued during their careers.
> Thirty-seven percent had at least one claim from residency, and
> there were an average of 2.6 claims per obstetrician. Sixty-two
> percent of these claims were from obstetrics as opposed to gynecol-
> ogy. The articles in this issue discuss various areas of perinatal
> medicine from the medical and legal perspectives, emphasizing
> those issues in maternal-fetal medicine that are the most frequent
> subjects of medical malpractice litigation.

**How Does a Physician Avoid Prescribing Drugs and
Medical Procedures That Have Reproductive
and Developmental Risks?**   233

Robert L. Brent

> The medicolegal climate in the United States has changed consider-
> ably in the past 50 years. This article provides practical tips that
> obstetricians and perinatologists can use to reduce the likelihood
> of being a defendant in malpractice litigation.

Congenital Disabilities and the Law   263

Robert Roth

> This article describes the evolution and stutter steps in the legal
> developments surrounding the controversial claims for "wrongful

conception," "wrongful birth," and "wrongful life." These claims arise from negligence in a failed vasectomy/tubal ligation resulting in an unwanted pregnancy and from negligence in failing to perform or properly interpret genetic testing resulting in the inability of parents to make an informed decision whether to terminate a pregnancy where a child would be, and ultimately is, born with serious genetic defects.

Informed Consent

Laurence B. McCullough and Frank A. Chervenak

Informed consent is an essential component of the practice of perinatal medicine because, as a process of communication and decision making, it should shape the relationship between the physician and pregnant woman and between the physician and the parents of a newborn child. This article provides an account of the physician's obligations in the informed consent process in terms of ethics and law.

Medical Legal Issues in Prenatal Diagnosis

Roger D. Klein and Maurice J. Mahoney

The capacity to diagnose fetal disease or abnormality continues to grow, especially in the genetic definition of the fetus. With this growth have come claims of medical malpractice that have mostly centered on a failure of informed consent. Failure may occur by omission or failed communication of pertinent information to the parents or by alleged error in the interpretation of diagnostic information. The usual claim against a physician or other provider is not that of causing damage or disease in the fetus but of causing a loss of opportunity to prevent conception or live birth of an infant who has an abnormality. Successful suits for "wrongful birth," brought by parents of an abnormal child, are common in many United States jurisdictions, but suits for "wrongful life," brought on behalf of the child, have usually been denied.

Medical Legal Issues in Obstetric Ultrasound

Frank A. Chervenak and Judith L. Chervenak

More than any other innovation, ultrasound has revolutionized the practice of obstetrics and gynecology in one generation. Unfortunately, there are medical legal risks of which all practitioners should be aware. This article discusses the general aspects of a medical negligence case as they relate to the performance of the obstetric ultrasound examination, summarizes the recommendations of the American College of Obstetricians and Gynecologists and the American Institute of Ultrasound in Medicine regarding the performance of these examinations, outlines potential areas of negligence, and discusses ways to avoid them.

delivery. A perspective on accusations relating to the failure to identify or to act on intrapartum asphyxia has been presented elsewhere in this issue. This article focuses on legal allegations that arise from the conduct of labor and the timing of delivery, independent of those related to fetal monitoring.

GOAL STATEMENT

The goal of *Clinics in Perinatology* is to keep practicing neonatologists and maternal-fetal medicine specialists up to date with current clinical practice in perinatology by providing timely articles reviewing the state of the art in patient care.

ACCREDITATION

The *Clinics in Perinatology* is planned and implemented in accordance with the Essential Areas and Policies of the Accreditation Council for Continuing Medical Education (ACCME) through the joint sponsorship of the University of Virginia School of Medicine and Elsevier. The University of Virginia School of Medicine is accredited by the ACCME to provide continuing medical education for physicians.

The University of Virginia School of Medicine designates this educational activity for a maximum of 60 *AMA PRA Category 1 Credits*™. Physicians should only claim credit commensurate with the extent of their participation in the activity.

The American Medical Association has determined that physicians not licensed in the US who participate in this CME activity are eligible for *AMA PRA Category 1 Credits*™.

Credit can be earned by reading the text material, taking the CME examination online at http://www.theclinics.com/home/cme, and completing the evaluation. After taking the test, you will be required to review any and all incorrect answers. Following completion of the test and evaluation, your credit will be awarded and you may print your certificate.

FACULTY DISCLOSURE/CONFLICT OF INTEREST

The University of Virginia School of Medicine, as an ACCME accredited provider, endorses and strives to comply with the Accreditation Council for Continuing Medical Education (ACCME) Standards of Commercial Support, Commonwealth of Virginia statutes, University of Virginia policies and procedures, and associated federal and private regulations and guidelines on the need for disclosure and monitoring of proprietary and financial interests that may affect the scientific integrity and balance of content delivered in continuing medical education activities under our auspices.

The University of Virginia School of Medicine requires that all CME activities accredited through this institution be developed independently and be scientifically rigorous, balanced and objective in the presentation/discussion of its content, theories and practices.

All authors/editors participating in an accredited CME activity are expected to disclose to the readers relevant financial relationships with commercial entities occurring within the past 12 months (such as grants or research support, employee, consultant, stock holder, member of speakers bureau, etc.). The University of Virginia School of Medicine will employ appropriate mechanisms to resolve potential conflicts of interest to maintain the standards of fair and balanced education to the reader. Questions about specific strategies can be directed to the Office of Continuing Medical Education, University of Virginia School of Medicine, Charlottesville, Virginia.

The authors/editors listed below have identified no professional or financial affiliations for themselves or their spouse/partner:
Isaac Blickstein, MD (Guest Editor); Robert L. Brent, MD, PhD, DSc (HON); Judith L. Chervenak, MD, JD (Guest Editor); Frank A. Chervenak, MD (Guest Editor); Wayne R. Cohen, MD; Carla Holloway (Acquisitions Editor); William M. Huang, MD; Roger D. Klein, MD, JD; Maurice J. Mahoney, MD, JD; Laurence B. McCullough, PhD; Robert Roth, BA, LLB; Barry S. Schifrin, MD; David E. Seubert, MD, JD; and, Randi Wasserman-Hoff, MD.

The authors/editors listed below identified the following professional or financial affiliations for themselves or their spouse/partner:
None

Disclosure of Discussion of non-FDA approved uses for pharmaceutical products and/or medical devices:
The University of Virginia School of Medicine, as an ACCME provider, requires that all faculty presenters identify and disclose any "off label" uses for pharmaceutical and medical device products. The University of Virginia School of Medicine recommends that each physician fully review all the available data on new products or procedures prior to instituting them with patients.

TO ENROLL

To enroll in the Clinics in Perinatology Continuing Medical Education program, call customer service at 1-800-654-2452 or visit us online at www.theclinics.com/home/cme. The CME program is available to subscribers for an additional fee of $195.00.

FORTHCOMING ISSUES

RECENT ISSUES

The Clinics are now available online!

Access your subscription at
www.theclinics.com

ELSEVIER
SAUNDERS

CLINICS IN
PERINATOLOGY

Clin Perinatol 34 (2007) xi–xiii

Preface

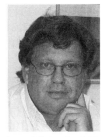

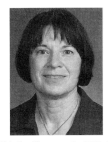

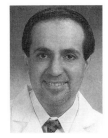

Isaac Blickstein, MD   Judith L. Chervenak, MD, JD   Frank A. Chervenak, MD

Guest Editors

The definition of medical malpractice is an act or omission by a health care provider that deviates from accepted standards of practice in the medical community and that causes injury to the patient. The specialty of perinatal medicine is among the top-ranking disciplines associated with malpractice claims in most developed countries. Perhaps the primary reason is that, by default, any pregnant woman expects to have a perfect child and to step out of the delivery room as healthy as she was before pregnancy. However, pregnancy and childbirth are essentially risky. When the maternal expectation does not concur with professional reality, dispute may arise. In addition, the overabundance of technology associated with prenatal diagnosis and the amount of sophistication available in perinatal medicine have led to the wrong popular perception of omnipotence. Often, a deviation from the expected perfect outcome is assumed to be a consequence of negligence.

As a result, the 2003 Annual Report from the National Practitioner Data Bank indicates that 16,764 medical malpractice payments were made due to obstetrics-related malpractice by physicians in the United States 1990 to 2003, with a mean and median medical malpractice payment due to obstetrics-related malpractice of $377,305 and $200,000, respectively. According to the same source, payments increased over the years, and among the 1255 medical malpractice payments made due to obstetrics-related malpractice in the United States 2003, the mean and median medical malpractice payment due to obstetrics-related malpractice were $475,880 and

doi:10.1016/j.clp.2007.04.002   *perinatology.theclinics.com*

$290,000, respectively. In total, $2,824,280,036 in payments was made for obstetrics-related primary malpractice acts or omissions in the United States 1990 to 1996.

These facts translate to increased malpractice insurance premiums, which in turn, have the potential to decrease future availability of specialist services. Despite these downsides, tort claims have a definite educational role by identifying weak points that need improvement and teaching the medical community about how to avoid negligence. On top of everything are lawyers who seek to provide compensation for damages occurring during the perinatal period because of alleged malpractice and negligence or to defend clinicians against such allegations. Collectively, the current medicolegal environment presents significant challenges to clinicians and lawyers.

In most lawsuits, cases with or without clear-cut malpractice are easily recognized. The problem is the "gray zone," which is unfortunately common in perinatal medicine. With these points in mind, our intention was neither to rewrite textbooks in perinatal medicine nor to provide guidelines for clinical practice. Instead, we wanted to identify and discuss the most common clinical situations that lead to legal disputes related to perinatal medicine to delineate the "gray zone," to focus on controversies, and to provide the contrasting perspective related to how a clinical situation is perceived by the practitioner and by the lawyer.

This issue of the *Clinics in Perinatology* presents an interdisciplinary discussion on medicolegal issues in perinatal medicine. First, a prelude overview on professional liability is presented. Second, basic concepts such as wrongful birth/life, informed consent, professional misconduct and ethics, and the expert witness are discussed. Third, we considered various aspects of the subspecialty such as fetal assessment and management of labor and delivery. Finally, we discuss the role of the placenta as a witness and error reduction and quality assurance in our practice.

The editors wish to thank all authors for the scholarly contributions and to Mrs. Carla Holloway—the production manager of this issue—for her continuous help and support.

Isaac Blickstein, MD
Department of Obstetrics and Gynecology
Kaplan Medical Center
76100 Rehovot, Israel

Hadassah-Hebrew University School of Medicine
Jerusalem, Israel

E-mail address: blick@netvision.net.il

Judith L. Chervenak, MD, JD
Heidell, Pittoni, Murphy & Bach, LLP
99 Park Avenue
New York, NY 10016, USA

New York University School of Medicine
550 First Avenue
New York, NY 10016, USA

E-mail address: jchervenak@hpmb.com

Frank A. Chervenak, MD
Department of Obstetrics and Gynecology
Joan and Sanford I. Weill Medical College of Cornell University
The New York Presbyterian Hospital
525 East 68th Street, Box 122
New York, NY 10021, USA

E-mail address: fac2001@med.cornell.edu

ELSEVIER
SAUNDERS

CLINICS IN
PERINATOLOGY

Clin Perinatol 34 (2007) 227–232

Overview of Professional Liability

Judith L. Chervenak, MD, JD[a,b]

[a]New York University School of Medicine, 550 First Avenue, New York, NY 10016, USA
[b]Heidell, Pittoni, Murphy & Bach, LLP, 99 Park Avenue, New York, NY 10016, USA

Scope of the problem

Eighty-nine percent of American College of Obstetricians and Gynecologists (ACOG) fellows responding to the 2006 Professional Liability Survey indicated that they had been sued during their careers. Thirty-seven percent had at least one claim from residency, and there were an average of 2.6 claims per obstetrician [1]. Sixty-two percent of these claims were from obstetrics as opposed to gynecology [1]. The survey, which covered claims opened or closed from January 1, 2003 through December 31, 2005, found that 31% were related to a neurologically impaired infant, whereas 16% were related to a stillbirth or a neonatal death [1]. In the articles that follow, the authors, some of whom are both physicians and lawyers, discuss various areas of perinatal medicine from the medical and legal perspectives, emphasizing those issues in maternal-fetal medicine that are the most frequent subjects of medical malpractice litigation.

Medical negligence

In the United States system, there are four elements that the plaintiff must prove to be successful in a claim for medical negligence: (1) a duty recognized by the law; (2) a failure on the part of the person to conform to the standard required; (3) a reasonably close connection between the conduct and the resulting injury, known as the "proximate or legal cause"; and (4) actual loss or damage to the interests of another [2]. The vast majority of these cases are brought in state court, and therefore the laws governing such issues as evidence, discovery, and statute of limitations can vary depending on the state. Because these are civil and not criminal cases, these elements must be proven by preponderance or 51% of the evidence [3].

E-mail address: jchervenak@hpmb.com

doi:10.1016/j.clp.2007.03.002 *perinatology.theclinics.com*

Most states require that an attorney submit an affirmation indicating that he has consulted with an expert who is qualified to provide an opinion as to whether there was a deviation from the standard of care and a causal relationship between that deviation and the damages to the plaintiff [4]. Although this expert is usually a physician, most often he is not of the same specialty or subspecialty as the defendant physician(s) and therefore may not be familiar with the particular specialty on which he has been asked to opine [2].

Duty

The duty to the patient is considered to be a contractual one that is not written but rather is implied from the actions of the parties when the physician–patient relationship is established [5]. Although most states have enacted Good Samaritan legislation, these statutes rarely apply to hospitalized patients [6]. The Emergency Medical Treatment and Active Labor Act ensures that those who seek care from an emergency department receive appropriate treatment and screening regardless of their ability to pay. Therefore, a legal obligation to care for a laboring patient can arise without the existence of a prior physician–patient relationship [7]. In some cases, the physician's duty can be expanded to include an obligation to future pregnancies and to include a duty to warn significant others [7].

Standard of care

The standard to which a physician is held is usually expressed as "the minimum knowledge, skill and care ordinarily possessed and employed by members of the profession in good standing" [2]. For those who hold themselves out to be specialists, the standard is modified accordingly. A single standard of care often does not exist, and if a physician's judgment is reasonable under the circumstances, he will not be held liable for a mistake in judgment. It should be recognized that this may "… permit mutually exclusive choices to be within the standard of care" [8].

If the jury is considered capable of determining whether the physician has met the applicable standard of care, the doctrine of *res ipsa loquitor* applies [5]. For example, if a physician leaves an instrument inside of an abdomen after surgery and that physician was in exclusive control of that instrument, a jury could find that such practice was below the accepted standard. In most medical malpractice cases, juries are deemed to need the assistance of an expert witness when determining the appropriate standard to apply. These expert witnesses are limited by the state of medical knowledge and practice at the time of the incident when opining on the appropriateness of the physician's actions [9]. In most legal cases, witnesses can only testify to that which they themselves have observed with their own senses to allow the jury to have some basis upon which to judge their credibility. In medical malpractice trials, however, experts are allowed to testify about events that they have not witnessed and to matters that are outside the general knowledge of most jurors, especially regarding causation of the injury.

Causation

For the plaintiffs to be successful, the plaintiffs must also show (1) that the deviation from the standard of care was the "proximate or legal cause of the injury" and (2) that the plaintiff sustained actual damages as a result [2]. Although experts are limited to the standards of medical practice that existed at the time of the alleged malpractice, causation testimony may include currently accepted theories that may explain whether any deviation from the standard of care caused the damage to the mother or infant in the case of an obstetrical claim [9].

Most jurisdictions require that there is a better than 50% probability that the alleged conduct caused the harm. This requirement is often not met when the patient has a pre-existing condition and alleges a lost opportunity for cure. In *Falcon v Memorial Hospital*, a Michigan Court held that a woman who suffered an amniotic fluid embolism could recover for negligent treatment even though there was testimony that her chances of survival were only 33% had she been given what was alleged to be proper treatment [10].

Challenges to expert testimony

In 1923, *Frye v U.S.* [11] was decided by a U.S. District Court. This Court, in attempting to determine whether testimony should be allowed, said that "just when scientific principle or discovery crosses the line between the experimental and demonstrable stages is difficult to define" but that when scientific testimony is offered, it "… must be sufficiently established to have gained general acceptance in the particular field in which it belongs." In 1993, the Supreme Court attempted to refine the criteria by which expert testimony should be evaluated in *Daubert v Merrill Dow* (which is discussed in the article by Brent elsewhere in this issue [12]). In Daubert, plaintiffs produced eight different expert witnesses who claimed to believe that Bendectin was teratogenic despite evidence in the medical literature that overwhelming documented the safety of the drug [13]. In excluding the plaintiffs' experts, the Court said that Courts should act as gatekeepers by determining if the proposed testimony is scientifically valid and if the proposed testimony "can properly be applied to the facts at issue." It set forth the following criteria: (1) whether the expert's technique or theory can be or has been tested; (2) whether the technique or theory has been subject to peer review and publication; (3) the known or potential rate or error of the technique or theory when applied; (4) the existence and maintenance of standards and controls; and 5) whether the technique or theory has been generally accepted in the scientific community [13]. This type of challenge to expert causation testimony can be made in the form of a summary judgment motion, a motion in limine before trial, or a motion to strike the testimony of the expert in question and to ask the Court for a directed verdict. The Court may hold a hearing before or during the trial outside the presence of the jury, during which the expert's testimony is challenged. In these cases, the defendant asks the Court to dismiss the case or to preclude plaintiff's expert from testifying because plaintiff's theory of causation is based upon an expert's opinion or theory that is not scientifically reliable.

In addition, a post-trial motion for relief can be made, as was done in *Lara v N.Y.C.H.H.C.,* 305 A.D.2d 106 (1st Dep't 2003) [14]. In Lara, the New York State Appellate Division upheld the dismissal of a case in which the plaintiff's expert opined that a slow bleed in the infant's brain led to the development of cerebral palsy. In doing so, the Court made clear that it would not accept a theory solely because the expert who was proffering that theory had a certain level of experience in a particular field.

Professional specialty societies, including ACOG and the American Association of Neurological Surgeons, have begun to censure or dismiss those experts among their members who they determined have violated certain ethical standards when giving testimony regarding standards of care or who have put forward spurious theories of causation in Court. ACOG has put forward the following criteria for expert witnesses [7]:

- They must possess a valid unrestricted medical license.
- They should be board certified with relevant training and clinical experience.
- They should have been clinically active in the relevant specialty for the previous 5 years, with participation in Continuing Medical Education (CME) relevant to the case.
- They should disclose the percentage of professional time they spend testifying in professional liability cases, the fee being paid, and the number of times they have testified for the defense and for the plaintiff.

To this end, ACOG has developed an Expert Witness Affirmation that an expert should be willing to sign indicating that he or she will be "truthful, impartial and fair, has relevant experience and is able to be nonjudgmental" and "that he/she would be willing to allow his/her testimony to be subjected to peer review" [7].

Other causes of action in obstetrical cases

Most United States jurisdictions recognize at least two other legal causes of action regarding birth-related injuries, which are more fully discussed in the article by Roth elsewhere in this issue. A wrongful birth action can be brought after negligent genetic counseling or negligent failure to diagnose a fetal defect or disease on behalf of the parents who seek to recover the extraordinary expenses of raising the impaired child whom they were denied the opportunity to abort [5]. A wrongful pregnancy action is brought on behalf of the parents in the case of a negligent sterilization procedure for the costs of having to raise a healthy but unplanned child. Most United States courts have rejected a wrongful life cause of action that is brought on behalf of a child who is born with a defect as result of negligent counseling or prenatal diagnosis and who argues that it would have been better not to have been born at all.

Impact of malpractice litigation in obstetrics

ACOG's 2006 Professional Liability Survey revealed that as a result of increased malpractice premium/insurance availability, 28.5% of obstetricians increased the number of Cesarean deliveries, 26.4% stopped offering vaginal birth after Cesarean, 25.6% decreased the number of high-risk patients, and 7.2% stopped practicing obstetrics altogether [1].

ACOG and many political groups support various methods of tort reform. Some of these initiatives are patterned after those in other countries, whereas others are attempts to uniquely improve the American system. Among the most common types of tort reform are (1) caps on damages, (2) making it more difficult to file a claim, (3) replacing litigation with another system such as a no-fault one, or (4) offering immunity to certain groups of providers from some types of suits [15].

It remains to be seen which of these strategies or in what combination reforms to the American system will lead to the optimal and most enduring solutions to the problems mentioned in this article. It is essential that obstetrician-gynecologists maintain professional integrity when dealing with professional liability issues [16].

References

[1] American College of Obstetrics and Gynecology. 2006 professional liability survey. Available at: www.acog.org. Accessed May 1, 2007.

[2] Prosser W, Keeton WP, Dobbs DB, et al. Prosser and Keeton on the law of torts. 5th edition. (MN): West Publishing Group; 1984. p. 187.

[3] Garner B, editors, Black's law dictionary, 7th edition. St. Paul (MN): West Group; 1999, p. 1201.

[4] Donohue RH. A defense attorney's perspective on medical negligence litigation. Clin Perinatol 2005;32:171.

[5] Furrow BR, Greaney TL, Johnson SH, et al. Health law: cases, materials and problems. 4th edition. St. Paul (MN): West Group; 2001. p. 189–90.

[6] American College of Obstetricians and Gynecologists. 2005 Legislative program: district II website. Available at: info@nyacog.org. Accessed May 1, 2007.

[7] American College of Obstetricians and Gynecologists. Professional liability and risk management, an essential guide for obstetrician-gynecologists. Washington DC: ACOG; 2005. p. 9–10.

[8] Schifrin BS. Malpractice issues in perinatal medicine: the United States perspective in fetal neonatal neurology & neurosurgery. 3rd edition. New York: Churchill Livingstone; 2001.

[9] Moore T, Gaier M. Medical malpractice. N Y Law J 2004;1.

[10] Falcon v Memorial Hospital, 462 N.W. 2d 44 (Mich. 1990).

[11] Frye v United States, 293 F. 1013 (D.C. Cir. 1923).

[12] Daubert v Merrel Dow Pharmaceuticals, Inc., 509 U.S. 579 (1993).

[13] Gebauer ME. The "what" and "how" of Daubert challenges to expert testimony under the new federal rule of Evidence 702, Pennsylvania Bar Quarterly. April 2002.

[14] Lara v N.Y.C.H.H.C., 305 A.D.2d 106 (1st Dept 2003).

[15] Association of Professors of Gynecology and Obstetrics. Medical-legal issues in obstetrics and gynecology. Washington, DC: Association of Professors of Gynecology and Obstetrics; 1994. p. 53–5.

[16] Chervenak FA, McCullough LB. Neglected ethical dimensions of the professional liability crisis. Am J Obstet Gynecol 2004;190(5):1198–200.

ELSEVIER
SAUNDERS

CLINICS IN
PERINATOLOGY

Clin Perinatol 34 (2007) 233–262

How Does a Physician Avoid Prescribing Drugs and Medical Procedures That Have Reproductive and Developmental Risks?

Robert L. Brent, MD, PhD, DSc (Hon)

Laboratory of Clinical and Environmental Teratology, Room 308, R/A, Alfred I. DuPont Hospital for Children, Box 269, Wilmington, DE 19899, USA

In 1967 I published an article titled the "Medicolegal Aspects of Teratology" in which I predicted the epidemic in malpractice litigation. This speculation was based on an influx of requests to evaluate the merits of what I characterized as nonmeritorious malpractice cases involving birth defects [1]. Even in the 1960s teratologists were aware that only a small percentage of birth defects were caused by drugs, chemicals, and physical agents [2–8]. In 2007 even more information is available to confirm this viewpoint (Table 1) [9–11]. Birth defects caused by drugs, chemicals, and physical agents account for a very small percentage of birth defects (see Table 1).

In the United States the medicolegal climate has changed considerably in the past 50 years. When I was appointed to the faculty at the Jefferson Medical College in Philadelphia in 1957, my malpractice premium was $50.00 per year. I am certain it is hard for many young obstetricians and perinatologists to believe that fact. But the climate has changed dramatically. Two reports of congenital malformations can put a historical perspective on the present malpractice climate in the United States.

The philosophy of some members of the legal profession and of the public is that someone must be responsible for personal damages that have been incurred. Historically, the father or mother of a malformed infant was open to ridicule, criticism, or even persecution [12–14]. Folklore and superstition dominated the field, and the causes of malformations were attributed to evil spirits, fornication with animals, lewd thoughts, or other immoral acts. Certainly, in the 1600s no one could have thought of receiving compensation for the birth of a malformed child. The following case presentation highlights

E-mail address: rbrent@nemours.org

0095-5108/07/$ - see front matter © 2007 Published by Elsevier Inc.
doi:10.1016/j.clp.2007.03.003

Table 1
Causes of human congenital malformations observed during the first year of life

Suspected cause	Percentage of total
Unknown	65–75
Polygenic	—
Multifactorial (gene–environment interactions)	—
Spontaneous errors of development	—
Synergistic interactions of teratogens	—
Genetic	15–25
Autosomal and sex-linked inherited genetic disease	—
Cytogenetic (chromosomal abnormalities)	—
New mutations	—
Environmental	10
Maternal conditions: alcoholism; diabetes; endocrinopathies; phenylketonuria; smoking and nicotine; starvation; nutritional deficits	4
Infectious agents: rubella, toxoplasmosis, syphilis, herpes simplex, cytomegalovirus, varicella-zoster, Venezuelan equine encephalitis, parvovirus B19	3
Mechanical problems (deformations): amniotic band constrictions; umbilical cord constraint; disparity in uterine size and uterine contents	1–2
Chemicals, prescription drugs, high-dose ionizing radiation, hyperthermia	<1

Data from Brent RL. Utilization of developmental basic science principles in the evaluation of reproductive risks from pre- and postconception environmental radiation exposures. Teratology 1999;59:182–4.

the ignorance and superstition that surrounded the birth of a malformed off-spring in the seventeenth century:

At a General Court held at New Haven on March 2, 1641, it transpired that on the preceding February 14,

> John Wakeman a planter and member of this church acquainted the magistrates that a sow of his which he had lately bought of Henry Browning, then with pigge, had now brought among divers liveing and rightly shaped pigs, one prodigious monster, which he then brought with him to be viewed and considered. The monster was come to the full growth as the other piggs for ought could be discerned, butt brought forth dead. Itt had no haire on the whole body, the skin was very tender and a reddish white collour like a childs; the head most straing, itt had butt one eye in the middle of the face, and thatt large an open, like some blemished eye of a man; over the eye the bottome of the foreheade which was like a childes, a thing of flesh grew forth and hung downe, itt was hollow, and like a man's instrument of generation. A nose, mouth and chinne deformed, butt nott much unlike a childs the neck and eares had also such resemblance.

This description is that of a typical cyclopean monster. The record continues,

> [A] strange impression was allso upon many that saw the monster, (therein guided by the neare resemblance of the eye) that one George Spencer, late

servant to the said Henry Browning, had beene actor in unnatureall and abominable filthynes with the sow–.

(It came out during the proceedings that Spencer actually had not been in the service of Browning at the critical time!)

The aforementioned George Spencer so suspected hath butt one eye for use, the other hath (as itt is called) a pearle in itt, is whitishy Y deformed, and his deformed eye being beheld and compared together with the eye of the monster, seamed to be as like as the eye in the glass to the eye in the face.

There is little doubt that George Spencer had a cataract in one eye. That he "had beene formerly notorious in the plantation for a prophane, lying scoffing and lewd speritt" surely did not help his situation.

Although professing innocence, he was committed to prison on February 24. In jail he was visited by some of the magistrates and other fellow-Puritans and under their strong moral suasion admitted to being guilty of the suspected crime but almost immediately revoked his confession. There followed, up to the final day of the drama, a succession of admissions and revocations; but although he impudently and with desperate imprecations "against himselfe denied all thatt he had formerly confessed," witnesses testified in court to his former admissions, and their word was accepted as evidence. The court then "judged the crime cappitall, and thatt the prisoner and the sow, according to Levit, 20 and 15, should be put to death—." And so, on April 8, 1642, "The sow being first slaine in his sight, he ended his course here. God opening his mouth before his death, to give him the glory of his rightousness, to the full satisfaction of all them present, butt in other respects leaving him a terrible example of divine justice and wrath" [15,16].

Spencer's case is a cruel example of injustice. Injustices continue to occur, although they may not be as extreme as the case of George Spencer. In a recent time, however, when injustice occurs, it trends to favor the afflicted or the malformed. The following case, which was decided in the 1960s, is a good example of up-to-date injustice. A pregnant woman was involved in an automobile accident and claimed that the accident was responsible for her child's having Down syndrome. In *Sinkler v Kneal*, "The plaintiffs filed a complaint containing four counts. In the first count plaintiff Nancy D. Sinkler claimed in her own right $100,000 damages for lacerations and contusions and shock to her nervous system which resulted in the birth of a Mongoloid child, Rebecca" [17]. The majority opinion of the court pertaining to the third count was reported September 26, 1960, several years after the genetic aspects of Down syndrome had been clarified [18–20]. The majority opinion clearly devoted its entire discussion to the question of whether an injured unborn had the right to recover damages in a negligence suit [17,21].

The majority decision did not address the important question whether the malformation and the automobile accident involving a pregnant woman were related. There is no question that the majority decision was accurate and sound with regard to the biologic concept that the fetus is a separate organism. The court, however, was grossly negligent in taking for granted an etiologic relationship between a pregnant woman's automobile accident and the subsequent birth of a child who had Down syndrome. It is obvious that a turnabout has occurred. The "malformed" offspring and his parents are no longer accused. On the contrary they have become the plaintiffs, seeking recompense and justice for the malformation and the "injured" family, when, in the eyes of a lawyer and his medical consultants, the mother or infant has been treated negligently during the pregnancy.

Along with cancer, psychiatric illness, and hereditary diseases, reproductive problems have been viewed throughout history as diseases of affliction (Fig. 1). Inherent in the reactions of most cultures is that these diseases represent punishments for misdeeds [12–14]. Regardless of the irrationality of this viewpoint, these feelings do exist. Ancient Babylonian writings recount tales of mothers being put to death because they delivered malformed infants. As previously cited, George Spencer was slain by the Puritans in New Haven in the seventeenth century, having been convicted of fathering a cyclopean pig because the Puritans were unable to differentiate between George Spencer's cataract and the malformed pig's cloudy cornea [21]. In modern times, some individuals who have reproductive problems reverse the historical perspective and blame others for the occurrence of their congenital malformations, infertility, abortions, and hereditary diseases [22]. They place the responsibility for their illness on environmental agents dispensed by their health care provider or used by their employer.

Reproductive problems alarm the public, the press, and some scientists to a greater degree than most other diseases. In fact, severely malformed children are disquieting to health care providers, especially those not experienced in dealing with these problems. No physician is comfortable informing a family that their child has been born without arms and legs. The objective evaluation of environmental causes of reproductive diseases is clouded by the emotional climate that surrounds these diseases, resulting

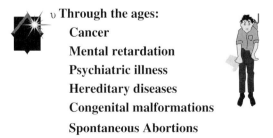

υ **Through the ages:**

Cancer

Mental retardation

Psychiatric illness

Hereditary diseases

Congenital malformations

Spontaneous Abortions

Fig. 1. Through the ages these diseases have been interpreted or considered by multiple cultures to be stigmatizing; punishments for misdeeds or sins. In modern times, environmental factors are thought to cause these diseases. Converting the guilt of the past into anger that is projected on others in our society sometimes leads to litigation.

in the expression of partisan positions that either diminish or magnify the environmental risks. These nonobjective opinions can be expressed by scientists, the laity, or the press [23]. It is the responsibility of every physician to be aware of the emotionally charged situation that is created when a family has a child with a birth defect. The inadvertent comment by a physician, nurse, resident, or student in attendance at the time of the child's delivery can have grave consequences for the physician and the family. Comments such as, "Oh, you had an X-ray during your pregnancy," or "You did not tell me that you were prescribed tetracycline while you were pregnant," can direct the patient's family to an attorney rather than to a teratology or genetic counselor.

How serious is the malpractice situation?

From the perspective of the perinatologist and the obstetrician, the answer is, "Very serious."

There were more than 210,000 closed claims reported to the data-sharing project of the Physician Insurer Association of America during a recent 20-year period [24]. Of the 28 medical specialties, the highest percentage of closed claims in which indemnity payments were made was ascribed to dentists, at 43%, with an average claim payment of $15,000.00. Obstetricians had the second-highest percentage of indemnity payments, at 36%, but the average claim payment was $110,000.00. Pediatricians account for 2.97% of these claims, making pediatrics the tenth among the 28 specialties in terms of the number of closed claims and sixteenth in terms of indemnity payment rate (28.13%). These figures include both settlements and lost lawsuits. The average cost to try a malpractice lawsuit is greater than the average settlement costs. Many nonmeritorious lawsuits are settled because it is cheaper for the insurance company to settle a case than to enter the courtroom and win.

Being a defendant in a malpractice lawsuit is an enervating, anxiety-provoking, time-consuming, and lengthy process. Some of these lawsuits last for years before they reach their conclusion [25]. The burden of the lawsuit can affect collegial relationships and the obstetrician's family life as well as his or her ability to carry out the practice of medicine. In many instances, the defendant feels like he or she is being treated like a criminal. Accusations and badgering in the deposition and even the courtroom can be distressing. It is an experience that every physician would rather avoid.

How does the obstetric community avoid product liability litigation?

The simple answer would be that the obstetrician can avoid product liability litigation by not prescribing drugs that have reproductive risks for the mother or developmental risks for the developing embryo or fetus. Table 2

Table 2
Proven human teratogens or embryotoxins: drugs, chemicals, milieus, and physical agents that
have resulted in human congenital malformations

Reproductive toxin	Alleged effects
Aminopterin, methotrexate	Growth retardation, microcephaly, meningomyelocele, mental retardation, hydrocephalus, and cleft palate
Androgens	Masculinization of the developing fetus can occur from androgens and high doses of some male-derived progestins
Angiotensin-converting enzyme inhibitors	Fetal hypotension syndrome in second and third trimester resulting in fetal kidney hypoperfusion and anuria, oligohydramnios, pulmonary hypoplasia, and cranial bone hypoplasia. No effect in the first trimester.
Antidepressants	Recent publications have implicated some of the SSRIs administered in the last trimester with postnatal neurobehavioral effects that are transient and whose long-term effects have not been determined. First-trimester exposures to some SSRIs have been reported to increase the risk of some congenital malformations, predominantly congenital heart disease. The results have not been consistent, but warnings have been issued.
Antituberculous therapy	Isoniazid and paraaminosalicylic acid have an increased risk for some CNS abnormalities.
Caffeine	Moderate caffeine exposure is not associated with birth defects; high exposures are associated with an increased risk of abortion but the data are inconsistent.
Chorionic villous sampling	Vascular disruption malformations (ie, limb-reduction defects)
Cobalt in hematemic multivitamins	Fetal goiter
Cocaine	Vascular disruptive type malformations in very low incidence; pregnancy loss
Corticosteroids	High exposures administered systemically have a low risk for cleft palate in some studies, but the epidemiologic studies are not consistent.

(*continued on next page*)

Table 2 (*continued*)

Reproductive toxin	Alleged effects
Cyclophosphamide and other chemotherapeutic agents and immunosuppressive agents (eg, cyclosporine, leflunomide)	Many chemotherapeutic agents used to treat cancer have a theoretical risk for producing malformations in the fetus when administered to pregnant women, especially because most of these drugs are teratogenic in animals, but the clinical data are not consistent. Many of these drugs have not been shown to be teratogenic, but the numbers of cases in the studies are small. Caution is the byword.
Diethylstilbestrol	Administration during pregnancy produces genital abnormalities, adenosis, and clear cell adenocarcinoma of vagina in adolescents. The last has a risk of 1:1000 to 1:10;000, but the other effects, such as adenosis, can be quite high.
Ethyl alcohol	Fetal alcohol syndrome consists of microcephaly, mental retardation, growth retardation, typical facial dysmorphogenesis, abnormal ears, small palpebral fissures.
Ionizing radiation	Radiation exposure above a threshold of 20 rad (0.2 Gy) can increase the risk for some fetal effects such as microcephaly or growth retardation, but the threshold for mental retardation is higher.
Insulin shock therapy	Insulin shock therapy, when administered to pregnant women, resulted in microcephaly, mental retardation.
Lithium therapy	Chronic usage for the treatment of manic-depressive illness has an increased risk for Ebstein's anomaly and other malformations, but the risk seems to be very low.
Minoxidil	This drug's promotion of hair growth was discovered because administration during pregnancy resulted in hirsutism in newborns.
Methimazole	Aplasia cutis has been reported to be increased in mothers administered this drug during pregnancy[a].
Methylene blue intra-amniotic instillation	Fetal intestinal atresia, hemolytic anemia, and jaundice in neonatal period. This procedure is no longer used to identify one twin.
Misoprostol	A low incidence of vascular disruptive phenomenon, such as limb-reduction defects and Mobius syndrome, has been reported in pregnancies in which this drug was used to induce an abortion.

(*continued on next page*)

Table 2 (*continued*)

Reproductive toxin	Alleged effects
Penicillamine (D-penicillamine)	This drug results in the physical effects referred to as "lathyrism," the results of poisoning by the seeds of the genus *Lathyrus*. It causes collagen disruption, cutis laxa, and hyperflexibility of joints. The condition seems to be reversible, and the risk is low.
Progestin therapy	Very high doses of androgen hormone–derived progestins can produce masculinization. Many drugs with progestational activity do not have masculinizing potential. None of these drugs have the potential for producing nongenital malformations.
Propylthiouracil	This drug and other antithyroid medications administered during pregnancy can result in an infant born with a goiter.
Radioactive isotopes	Tissue- and organ-specific damage depends on the radioisotope element and distribution (ie, high doses of Iodine-131 administered to a pregnant woman can cause fetal thyroid hypoplasia after the eighth week of development).
Retinoids	Systemic retinoic acid, isotretinoin, and etretinate can cause increased risk of CNS, cardioaortic, ear, and clefting defects such as mMicrotia, anotia, thymic aplasia, other branchial arch and aortic arch abnormalities, and certain congenital heart malformations.
Retinoids, topical	Topical administration is very unlikely to have teratogenic potential, because teratogenic serum levels cannot be attained by topical exposure to retinoids.
Streptomycin	Streptomycin and a group of ototoxic drugs can affect the eighth nerve and interfere with hearing; it is a relatively low-risk phenomenon. Children are less sensitive than adults to the ototoxic effects of these drugs.
Sulfa drugs and vitamin K	These drugs can produce hemolysis in some subpopulations of fetuses.
Tetracycline	This drug produces bone and teeth staining, it does not increase the risk of any other malformations.

(*continued on next page*)

Table 2 (*continued*)

Reproductive toxin	Alleged effects
Thalidomide	This drug results in an increased incidence of deafness, anotia, preaxial limb-reduction defects, phocomelia, ventricular septal defects, and gastrointestinal atresias. The susceptible period is from the twenty-second to the thirty-sixth day after conception.
Trimethorpin	This drug was used frequently to treat urinary tract infections and has been linked to an increased incidence of neural tube defects. The risk is not high, but it is biologically plausible because of the drug's effect on lowering folic acid levels, which has resulted in neurologic symptoms in adults taking this drug.
Vitamin A	The malformations reported with the retinoids have been reported with very high doses of vitamin A (retinol). Dosages to produce birth defects would have to be in excess of 25,000 to 50,000 units/d.
Vitamin D[a]	Large doses given in vitamin D prophylaxis may be involved in the etiology of supravalvular aortic stenosis, elfin faces, and mental retardation.
Warfarin and warfarin derivatives	Early exposure during pregnancy can result in nasal hypoplasia, stippling of secondary epiphysis, intrauterine growth retardation. Central nervous system malformations can occur in late pregnancy exposure because of bleeding.
Anticonvulsants Diphenylhydantoin	Treatment of convulsive disorders increases the risk of the fetal hydantoin syndrome, consisting of facial dysmorphology, cleft palate, ventricular septal defect, and growth and mental retardation.
Trimethadione and paramethadione	Treatment of convulsive disorders with these drugs increases the risk of characteristic facial dysmorphology, mental retardation, V-shaped eyebrows, low-set ears with anteriorly folded helix, high-arched palate, irregular teeth, CNS anomalies, and severe developmental delay.
Valproic acid	Treatment of convulsive disorders with this drug increases the risk of spina bifida, facial dysmorphology, and autism.
Carbamazepine	Treatment of convulsive disorders with this drug increases the risk facial dysmorphology.

(*continued on next page*)

Table 2 (*continued*)

Reproductive toxin	Alleged effects
Chemicals	
Carbon monoxide poisoning	Central nervous system damage has been reported with very high exposures, but the risk seems to be low[a].
Lead	Very high exposures can cause pregnancy loss; intrauterine teratogenesis is not established at very low exposures below 20 μg/% in the serum of pregnant mothers.
Gasoline addiction embryopathy	Facial dysmorphology, mental retardation
Methyl mercury	Minamata disease consists of cerebral palsy, microcephaly, mental retardation, blindness, and cerebellum hypoplasia. Other epidemics have occurred from adulteration of wheat with mercury-containing chemicals that are used to prevent grain spoilage. Present environmental levels of mercury are unlikely to represent a teratogenic risk, but reducing or limiting the consumption of carnivorous fish has been suggested to avoid exceeding the maximum permissible exposure recommended by the Environmental Protection Agency, an exposure level far below the level at which the toxic effects of mercury are seen
Polychlorinated biphenyls	Poisoning has occurred from adulteration of food products (" Cola-colored babies," CNS effects, pigmentation of gums, nails, teeth, and groin; hypoplastic deformed nails; intrauterine growth retardation; abnormal skull calcification). The threshold exposure has not been determined, but it is unlikely to be teratogenic at the present environmental exposures.
Toluene addiction embryopathy	Facial dysmorphology, mental retardation
Embryonic and fetal infections	
Cytomegalovirus infection	Retinopathy, CNS calcification, microcephaly, mental retardation
Rubella	Deafness, congenital heart disease, microcephaly, cataracts, mental retardation
Herpes simplex	Fetal infection, liver disease, death
HIV	Perinatal HIV infection
Parvovirus infection, B19	Stillbirth, hydrops
Syphilis	Maculopapular rash, hepatosplenomegaly, deformed nails, osteochondritis at joints of extremities, congenital neurosyphilis, abnormal epiphyses, chorioretinitis
Toxoplasmosis	Hydrocephaly, microphthalmia, chorioretinitis, mental retardation

(*continued on next page*)

Table 2 (continued)

Reproductive toxin	Alleged effects
Varicella zoster	Skin and muscle defects; intrauterine growth retardation; limb reduction defects, CNS damage (very low increased risk)
Venezuelan equine encephalitis	Hydranencephaly; microphthalmia; destructive CNS lesions; luxation of hip
Maternal disease states	
Corticosteroid-secreting endocrinopathy	Mothers who have Cushing's disease can have infants with hyperadrenocortism, but anatomic malformations do not seem to be increased.
Iodine deficiency	Can result in embryonic goiter and mental retardation
Intrauterine problems of constraint and vascular disruption	These defects are more common in multiple-birth pregnancies, pregnancies with anatomic defects of the uterus, placental emboli, or amniotic bands. Possible birth defects include club feet, limb-reduction defects, aplasia cutis, cranial asymmetry, external ear malformations, midline closure defects, cleft palate and muscle aplasia, cleft lip, omphalocele, and encephalocele)
Maternal androgen endocrinopathy (adrenal tumors)	Masculinization
Maternal diabetes	Caudal and femoral hypoplasia, transposition of great vessels, and other malformations
Maternal folic acid in reduced amounts	An increased incidence of neural tube defects
Maternal phenylketonuria	Abortion, microcephaly, and mental retardation; very high risk in untreated patients
Maternal starvation	Intrauterine growth restriction, abortion, neural tube defects (Dutch famine experience)
Tobacco smoking	Abortion, intrauterine growth restriction, stillbirth
Zinc deficiency[a]	Neural tube defects[a]

Abbreviation: CNS, central nervous system.
[a] Controversial.

describes the known agents that increase reproductive and developmental risks [9–11,26]. Unfortunately, the situation is not so straightforward. In many lawsuits alleging that congenital malformations were the result of a drug exposure, the allegation was incorrect (Box 1).

Progestational drugs

The largest number of product liability congenital malformation lawsuits that involved the obstetric community erroneously alleged that progestational

---

Box 1. Agents erroneously alleged to have caused human malformations

Bendectin: Alleged to cause numerous types of birth defects including limb-reduction defects, heart malformations, and many other malformations

Diagnostic ultrasonography: No significant hyperthermia, therefore no reproductive effects

Electromagnetic fields: Alleged to cause abortion, cancer, and birth defects

Progestational drugs: Alleged to cause numerous types of nongenital birth defects, including limb-reduction defects, heart malformations, and many other malformations

---

drugs were responsible for the occurrence of congenital malformations. Frequently, obstetricians were the physician defendants in these cases. Numerous lawsuits were filed or went to trial involving the progestational drugs, alleging that they were responsible for the occurrence of congenital heart disease or limb-reduction defects. In 1977 the Food and Drug Administration (FDA) placed a black box warning in the label of progestational drugs indicating that these drugs were associated with the occurrence of congenital heart disease and limb-reduction defects [27]. The warning was placed because several publications reported an association of progestational drugs and limb-reduction defects, congenital heart disease, and a few other malformations [28–37]. In 1999, 22 years after the black box warning, the FDA removed the warning [38,39].

Many of the lawsuits were decided in favor of the plaintiffs, although the majority of the lawsuits was decided in favor of the defendants. Irresponsible experts were one of the key contributors the plaintiffs' success in some of these lawsuits [23]. Obstetricians had to sit through lengthy trials, away from their family and practice, to defend themselves against an allegation that was totally erroneous. In 1977 extensive literature indicated that it was most unlikely that progestational drugs could produce nongenital malformations. In 1981 Wilson and Brent [40] published an extensive review and analysis of the allegation that progestational drugs could produce nongenital malformations and concluded that the allegation was incorrect. Other publications were in agreement [41,42], but 22 years elapsed before the warning was removed [27,39].

Bendectin

Another drug, Bendectin, was prescribed commonly by obstetricians for the treatment of nausea and vomiting of pregnancy. Thousands of lawsuits alleged that Bendectin was a teratogen, although Bendectin was the only drug approved by the FDA for the treatment of nausea and vomiting of pregnancy. During the 1970s, when Bendectin was used most frequently, it was prescribed to 30% of pregnant women. There are approximately 4,000,000 births each year in the United States, and the background incidence of major birth defects is 3% (Table 3). Therefore expected background incidence of birth defects would be 120,000; 36,000 newborns who had congenital anomalies would have been exposed to Bendectin each year. This prevalence was a bonanza for some plaintiff attorneys, because a jury might interpret these numbers as representing an epidemic of birth defects. The 36,000 birth defects, however, is exactly the expected background incidence of birth defects in the Bendectin-exposed group. This medication was studied extensively, and the allegation had no merit [43–53]. After 20 years of litigation, not a single Bendectin lawsuit was decided on behalf of the plaintiffs [49,50,53]. The medication was removed from the market in 1982, however, because the cost of litigation and negligence insurance was greater than the gross sales of the medication. The frequency of hospital admissions for nausea and vomiting of pregnancy doubled because Bendectin was not available, and physicians were reluctant to prescribe any medication for fear of litigation [51–53]. The numerous negative aspects of the Bendectin saga included (1) the loss of an approved medication for the treatment of nausea and vomiting of pregnancy, (2) the reluctance of many obstetricians to use any medication to treat nausea and vomiting of pregnancy, (3) the increase in hospital admissions for the treatment of nausea and vomiting of pregnancy [52], and (4) the waste of time and expenses to the courts of litigating nonmeritorious lawsuits.

Table 3
Frequency of reproductive risks in the human

Reproductive risk	Frequency
Immunologically and clinically diagnosed spontaneous abortions per 10^6 conceptions	350,000
Clinically recognized spontaneous abortions per 10^6 pregnancies	150,000
Genetic diseases per 10^6 births	110,000
Multifactorial or polygenic (genetic–environmental interactions)	90,000
Dominantly inherited disease	10,000
Autosomal and sex-linked genetic disease	1200
Cytogenetic (chromosomal abnormalities)	5000
New mutations	3000
Major congenital malformations per 10^6 births	30,000
Prematurity per 10^6 births	40,000
Fetal growth retardation per 10^6 births	30,000
Stillbirths/10^6 pregnancies (>20 weeks)	2000–20,900
Infertility	7% of couples

This plethora of litigation did have one major beneficial outcome, however. The Supreme Court rendered the famous Daubert decision as part of the litigation activities. It permitted jurists to disqualify the testimony of expert witnesses who used methodologic procedures that are not accepted and approved by the scientific community to reach their opinion [48]. The courts rejected the testimony of several of the plaintiffs' experts involved in the Daubert decision. This small group of irresponsible medical and scientific experts contributed negatively to the welfare of the obstetric patients in the United States [23,49,54].

This review of the progestational drug and Bendectin litigation is a reminder that lawsuits on behalf of a child who has congenital malformations can be instituted regardless of whether the allegation has scientific or medical merit. There are, however, drugs that can harm the developing embryo if administered at a sensitive period of embryonic development and at exposures high enough to affect the developing embryo or fetus deleteriously. This extensive list of potential embryo toxic agents is listed in Table 2. Box 1 lists some of the agents that have been involved in litigation that have not been demonstrated to affect the embryo deleteriously at their acceptable exposure.

These tables are simply lists that can be misused if one does not pay attention to the importance of timing and dose. For example, thalidomide is a known and proven teratogen, but if 1 mg were administered during the sensitive period of development, rather than the usual dose of 50 mg or greater, there would be no effect on the exposed embryo. Likewise, 50 mg of thalidomide administered during the sixth month of gestation never would result in the malformations observed in the typical thalidomide syndrome, because the sensitive period is so limited (Table 4).

Table 4
Developmental stage sensitivity to thalidomide-induced limb-reduction defects in the human

Days from conception for induction of defects	Limb-reduction defects
21–26	Thumb aplasia
22–23	Microtia, deafness
23–34	Hip dislocation
24–29	Amelia, upper limbs
24–33	Phocomelia, upper limbs
25–31	Preaxial aplasia, upper limbs
27–31	Amelia, lower limbs
28–33	Preaxial aplasia, lower limbs; phocomelia, lower limbs; femoral hypoplasia; girdle hypoplasia
33–36	Triphalangeal thumb

Data from Brent RL, Holmes LB. Clinical and basic science lessons from the thalidomide tragedy: what have we learned about the causes of limb defects? Teratology 1988; 38:244.

Anticonvulsants

Another example pertains to the administration of anticonvulsants to pregnant women because of the frequency with which anticonvulsants are administered. Diphenylhydantoin, when administered throughout pregnancy, increases the risk of congenital malformations that include facial dysmorphogenesis, microcephaly, decreased cognition, digital hypoplasia, and ventricular septal defects [55]. These malformations do not occur frequently, and the physician administering the drugs often is faced with a dilemma as to whether to continue the medication, reduce the medication, or discontinue use of the anticonvulsant during pregnancy. If, for example, a pregnant woman is in an automobile accident and sustains a head injury, the consulting neurosurgeon might prescribe one dose of 200 mg of phenytoin. It is unlikely that this single dose will result in the phenytoin embryopathy. This future mother, however, has a 3% risk of delivering a baby with congenital malformations. One can imagine how an irresponsible expert might testify if this mother delivers a child who has congenital malformations.

It is impossible to discuss each of the drugs in Table 2 and describe the circumstances when the embryo is or is not at risk. Publications dealing with the subject of teratogenic drugs, chemicals, and physical agents and the genetic causes of congenital malformations can be useful to clinicians for evaluating the risks of environmental toxicants [9–11,26,56–62].

Principles of counseling obstetric or perinatology patients about the risks of pregnancy and the therapy that may be necessary for the patient's care

Predicting the developmental risks of a pregnancy

Patients frequently ask obstetricians or perinatologists whether a particular preconception or postconception environmental exposure represented a risk for their developing embryo or fetus. For example, a pregnant patient might ask whether the chest radiograph that occurred early in her pregnancy could result in a newborn who had birth defects. The most appropriate answer would be:

> A chest radiograph does not expose the embryo to a harmful dose of radiation. The radiation exposure is so low that even the same exposure to your uterus would not increase your risk for having a child with birth defects. You must realize, however, that even if you have no personal or family history of reproductive or developmental problems, you began your pregnancy with a 3% risk for birth defects and a 15% risk for miscarriage.

This information should be communicated verbally and also be noted in the patient's medical chart. The obstetrician and perinatologist must be careful not to provide verbal guarantees concerning the outcome of the pregnancy (eg, "You have nothing to worry about"; "The baby will be fine."). In an effort to quell the patient's anxiety, the physicians may provide misinformation, because physicians cannot prevent the background incidence of developmental problems.

Understanding the principles of teratology to determine developmental risks

Five principles of teratology are useful for evaluating reproductive and developmental risks. These principles can assist clinicians in evaluating risks and in determining the significance of developmental effects in newborns and children that they have delivered [9–11,26]. When evaluating studies dealing with the reproductive effects of any environmental agent, important principles should guide the analysis of human and animal reproductive studies. Paramount to this evaluation is the application of the basic science principles of teratology and developmental biology [9–11,63]. These principles are as follows:

1. Exposure to teratogens follows a toxicologic dose–response curve. There is a threshold below which no teratogenic effect will be observed; as the dose of the teratogen is increased, both the severity and frequency of reproductive effects increase (Table 5).
2. The embryonic stage of exposure is critical in determining what deleterious effects will be produced and whether any of these effects can be produced by a known teratogen. Some teratogenic effects have a broad and others have a very narrow period of sensitivity. The most sensitive

Table 5
Stochastic and threshold dose-response relationships of diseases produced by environmental agents

Relationship	Pathology	Site	Diseases	Risk	Effect
Stochastic phenomena	Damage to a single cell may result in disease	DNA	Cancer mutation	Some risk exists at all dosages; at low exposures the hypothetical risk is below the spontaneous risk.	The incidence of the disease increases with the dose, but the severity and nature of the disease remain the same.
Threshold phenomena	Multi-cellular injury	High variation in etiology, affecting many cells and organ processes	Malformation, growth retardation, death, chemical toxicity, and others	No increased risk below the threshold dose	Both the severity and incidence of the disease increase with dose.

Data from Brent RL. The irresponsible expert witness: a failure of biomedical graduate education and professional accountability. Pediatrics 1982;70:754–62.

stage for the induction of mental retardation from ionizing radiation is from the eighth to the fifteenth week of pregnancy, a lengthy period. Thalidomide's period of sensitivity is approximately 2 weeks (see Table 4) [64].

3. Even the most potent teratogenic agent cannot produce every malformation.

4. Most teratogens have a limited group of congenital malformations that result after exposure during a critical period of embryonic development. This limited group of malformations is referred to as the syndrome that describes the agent's teratogenic effects.

5. Although a group of malformations may suggest the possibility of certain teratogens, they cannot confirm the causal agent definitively, because some teratogenic syndromes mimic genetic syndromes. On the other hand, the presence of certain malformations can eliminate the possibility that a particular teratogenic agent was responsible because those malformations have not been demonstrated to be part of the syndrome or because the production of that malformation is not biologically plausible for the particular alleged teratogen.

Determining whether an environmental agent has developmental or reproductive effects at the exposure to which the population is exposed

Evidence supporting or refuting the allegation that an environmental agent has reproductive or developmental effects at the typical human exposures comes from several areas of investigation [40,49,65]:

1. Consistency. Consistent findings in a number of epidemiologic studies in which statistical associations for a spectrum or group of developmental effects or specific reproductive effects are found in several studies

2. Secular trend analysis. Secular trend analysis can be used when a large percentage of the population has been exposed as with the progestational drugs or Bendectin. Changes in exposure caused by a reduction or cessation of prescribing may or may not alter the incidence of developmental or reproductive effects.

3. Animal reproductive studies. These studies are very useful in determining whether findings in epidemiologic studies can be confirmed in animal reproductive or developmental studies. Every environmental agent that has been confirmed to be a human teratogen or reproductive toxin has been found to be teratogenic in an animal model. When this confirmation cannot be accomplished, reproductive and developmental scientists are somewhat concerned about the validity of the causal relationship in the epidemiologic studies.

4. Dose–response relationships and pharmacokinetic studies comparing human and animal metabolism. One important aspect of modern preclinical testing protocols is that serum and/or tissue levels of the drug or chemical are determined in both the animal model and in humans. If reproductive and developmental effects occur in the animal model

at serum or tissue levels that occur in humans, there should be concern about the safety of the drug or chemical.

5. Biologic plausibility. This concept is important, because in some instances scientific considerations can support or refute an allegation of the reproductive or developmental toxicity. For example, the original epidemiology studies involving progestational drugs reported that epidemiologic studies showed an increased incidence of congenital heart disease but no increase in the incidence of limb-reduction defects. In other studies there was an increased incidence of limb-reduction defects but no increase in the incidence of congenital heart disease. Those findings, in themselves, should have refuted the allegation. Second, progestational drugs function by attaching to sex steroid receptors. Early in embryonic development there are no sex steroid receptors in the developing heart and limb buds. Biologic plausibility involves consideration of
   a. Mechanisms
   b. Receptor studies
   c. Nature of the malformations
   d. Mechanism of action
   d. Teratology principles

It should be apparent that determining the reproductive risks of an exposure during pregnancy or the origin of a child's congenital malformations is not a simple process. It involves a careful analysis of the medical and scientific literature pertaining to the reproductive toxic effects of exogenous agents in humans and animals as well as an evaluation of the exposure and biologic plausibility of an increased risk or a causal connection between the exposure and a child's congenital malformation. It also involves a review of the scientific literature pertaining to genetic and environmental causes of the malformations in question. An abridged or superficial evaluation based on incomplete analyses is not acceptable.

What circumstances stimulate negligence lawsuits?

Certain circumstances seem to stimulate negligence lawsuits in cases of birth defects [1,23,25,51,66]:

1. A plaintiff who generates sympathy, a defense expert who frequently is unable to be certain of the cause of the child's birth defect, and a plaintiff expert who is certain
2. Neurobehavioral effects, mental retardation, cerebral palsy
3. Miscarriage
3. A high proportion of exposures in the population at risk
4. A scientific topic that has attracted junk scientists as experts
5. Jurisdictions or geographic areas that are known to favor plaintiff verdicts
6. A litigation subject that has become attractive to number of law firms

7. A new area (drug) for which little data are available and therefore hypotheses without data can be generated
8. Vaccinations given during pregnancy

Clinical situations in which the obstetrician or perinatologist is the primary provider and the therapy and/or diagnostic tests may represent potential or hypothetical reproductive and developmental risks

It is impossible to discuss all the medications and pre- and postconception therapies that obstetricians might use to care for their patients. The following is a short list of categories of therapy for which patients have filed lawsuits alleging that the obstetrician's or perinatologist's treatment resulted in harm to the fetus:

1. Nausea and vomiting of pregnancy
2. Treatment of hypertension
3. Treatment of psychiatric problems (depression, anxiety)
4. Exposure to various forms of "radiation"
5. Medications and therapy to manage premature labor
6. Treatment of infections
7. Immunizations
8. Diagnostic radiologic studies
9. Diagnostic ultrasonography

Treating nausea and vomiting of pregnancy

In the 1960s there was an increase in the number of lawsuits involving malformed children and their families as plaintiffs [1]. Many of the lawsuits involved an antinausea medication, such as meclizine. The first meclizine lawsuit with which I was acquainted occurred in the late 1960s and involved a child who had ectrodactyly, ectodermal dysplasia, and cleft palate—EEC syndrome, which is a genetic disease. Scientists from a prestigious university and the from National Institutes of Health testified that meclizine caused this child's defect; of course, the defect, in fact, was present at the time of conception, before there was any exposure to the medication.

Bendectin containing doxylamine succinate, dicyclomine, and pyridoxine was listed as appropriate for the treatment of nausea and vomiting of pregnancy. The FDA approved labeling for Bendectin as the only drug formerly recommended for the treatment of nausea and vomiting in pregnant women.

Benefits of effective treatment

It is obvious that clinical, psychologic, and social benefits result from any effective therapy that reduces the symptoms of nausea and vomiting in pregnant women. The benefits include

1. Symptomatic improvement and comfort
2. Preventing the progression of symptoms to necessitate hospitalization

3. Optimal nutrition for mother and fetus
4. Decreased risk of some pregnancy complications
5. Psychologic benefits
6. Decrease absenteeism for working mothers
7. Decreased difficulty in managing the home and family

Medical risks of therapeutic intervention

The medical risks of any therapy have two implications. The first is that the therapy may be unacceptable to the patient or may represent a medical risk that is unacceptable to the physician and the patient. In other circumstances the theoretic risk of a new therapy could be more significant than the benefit of relieving the nausea and vomiting. Some of these risks, if they occur, could lead to litigation. The most serious medicolegal risk is the occurrence of embryonic and fetal malformations.

Legal risks of therapeutic intervention

Because many of the therapies for nausea and vomiting of pregnancy are relatively new, there are minimal data on which to base an evaluation of the risk of reproductive effects. Unfortunately, attorneys can be creative in generating hypotheses and obtaining witnesses who are willing to support hypotheses that implicate the therapy as having teratogenic potential [23,25]. Even when therapies such as acupressure, hypnosis, psychotherapy, or psychologic conditioning seem to be very unlikely to harm the fetus, that unlikelihood does not prevent a lawsuit from being initiated if a severely malformed fetus results from a pregnancy. Therefore, the best protection for the patient, the physician, the manufacturer of a drug, or the developer of a therapeutic technique is to have abundant data that indicate that the therapy has no measurable harmful effects on the developing embryo or fetus or on pregnant women. Unfortunately, only one therapy that fits these criteria, and that is Bendectin (10 mg each of doxylamine succinate and pyridoxine). Twelve cohort studies and numerous case-control studies, involving more than 13,000 patients, indicate that Bendectin does not represent a measurable risk to the developing mother or fetus. Furthermore, the animal studies and in vitro studies support this conclusion [49,50,53]. No other treatment of nausea and vomiting during pregnancy has the demonstrated low-risk record of Bendectin. Unfortunately, this medication is no longer sold in the United States, but it is sold in Canada under a proprietary name [67]. It has the same constituents as Bendectin (10 mg of pyridoxine and 10 mg of doxylamine succinate).

In 1999 the FDA published a statement in the Federal Register that summarizes the FDA's opinion on the lack of teratogenicity of Bendectin [68]. In summary:

> The Food and Drug Administration has determined that the drug product Bendectin, a tablet composed of pyridoxine hydrochloride, 10 mg, and doxylamine succinate, 10 mg, for the prevention of nausea during pregnancy,

was not withdrawn from sale for reasons of safety or effectiveness. This determination will permit FDA to approve abbreviated new drug applications for the combination product pyridoxine hydrochloride, 10 mg, and doxylamine succinate, 10 mg, tablets.

Treatment of hypertension during pregnancy

Toxemia of pregnancy, renal hypertension, lupus hypertension, idiopathic "essential" hypertension, and other causes of hypertension represent serious medical problems during pregnancy. Fortunately, there are numerous excellent medications to treat high blood pressure. Two classes of medications, however, have serious, deleterious effects on fetal development [69–72]. Fetal exposure during the second and third trimester to angiotensin-converting enzyme inhibitors or the angiotensin II receptor blockers may produce severe fetal hypotension, oligohydramnios, pulmonary hypoplasia, fetal and neonatal renal failure, and decreased calcification of the skull. If the fetus survives, death can occur postnatally from renal or pulmonary failure. Some children survive after renal transplantation. Animal studies support the clinical impression that the second and third trimester are the vulnerable period when the drugs do their damage and that exposure during early organogenesis does not seem to have any detrimental effect from. A recent article by Cooper and colleagues [73] indicates that there is an increased risk of congenital malformations with first trimester exposures, but the animal studies and other epidemiologic studies do not support these findings.

Treatment of psychiatric problems (depression, anxiety) during pregnancy

Many drugs that are used for the treatment of psychiatric disorders demonstrate transient behavioral effects in newborns whose mothers received these medications before delivery of the infant. Transient irritability, jitteriness, and depression may be manifested, depending on the primary effects of the medication. Very few of these drugs have been reported to be associated with reproductive or developmental effects, although some of the anticonvulsants that have psychopharmacologic therapeutic effects (eg, diphenylhydantoin, valproic acid, carbamazepine, phenobarbital) have been associated with an increased risk of birth defects (see Table 2).

Recently the selective serotonin receptor reductase inhibitors (SSRIs) have been studied for first-trimester teratogenic effects, and paroxetine was reported to be associated with an increased risk of congenital heart disease [74,75]. These findings have not been consistent, however, because there are studies that do not confirm these findings [76,77]. The few animal studies that have been reported do not find teratogenic effects [78]. The increased teratogenic risks following first-trimester exposure to SSRIs has yet to be resolved, although the FDA and the companies involved have issued warnings about the potential teratogenicity of SSRIs.

Radiation exposures

The public and some health care providers have concerns about new diagnostic radiation modalities using radiographs and radionuclides. Some physicians and many patients assume that these new procedures involve much higher exposures and much higher risks. It is important that all the new procedures and their embryonic risks be placed in proper perspective. These procedures include

> CT scans and positron emission tomograph scans
> MRI studies (Many patients believe that X-rays are involved in these studies, which is not true. The electromagnetic fields used in MRI studies are non-ionizing forms of radiation.)
> Diagnostic scans using radionuclides for studying the location of a pulmonary embolus, the presence of gallbladder disease, cardiac perfusion, cardiac stress test, areas of bone inflammation or injury, thyroid function, liver function, renal perfusion, lung perfusion, and other conditions

There are misconceptions concerning the reproductive and developmental risks of low exposures of ionizing radiation from occupational exposures and airplane travel, especially the magnitude of the risk from solar flares. Health care providers who work in medical or research fields have exaggerated concerns about the reproductive or developmental risks of their on-the-job exposures. Among the most common concerns are those of dental technicians who perform the dental radiographic examinations in a dentist's office and nurses and operating room assistants who are in proximity to fluoroscopes or brachytherapy procedures in the operating room.

Pregnant patients receiving radiation therapy for the treatment of cancer or other serious diseases are in a special category. If the fetus is in the therapeutic beam, it is likely that the treatment will be harmful to the developing embryo. The developmental risks also can be increased in pregnant women receiving therapeutic doses of radionuclides.

Concern about the risk of infertility or genetic disease in their children from preconception radiation exposure of the ovaries or testicles has been increasing among patients contacting the Health Physics Ask the Expert Website.

The public and some health care providers have old and new concerns about the risks of harm to the embryo from non-ionizing "radiation" because of misconceptions about the risks that can be ascribed to the many forms of non-ionizing radiation. Although addressing these issues may seem unnecessary, these exposures can generate as much concern and anxiety as the exposures to ionizing radiation that do represent a real risk to the embryo. These concerns have been communicated frequently to the Health Physics Society Website, Ask The Expert [66,79–82]. Matters of concern include

Diagnostic ultrasound procedures that expose the embryo or expose other parts of the body of a pregnant woman

Exposure to electromagnetic fields from power lines, house appliances, electric commuter trains

Exposure to or proximity to microwave communication antennae for fire departments, police departments, ambulance services, or cellular telephone communications

Exposure to personal cellular telephones (birth defects in their embryo and cancer in themselves)

Visiting a tanning salon while pregnant

Laser hair removal from the abdomen or thigh of pregnant patients

Use of an ultrasound sonicator for preparing tissue or cleaning jewelry

Use of a hair dryer, computer, cellular telephone, or microwave oven

Working in an office or other site in proximity to a microwave dish

Walking through a metal detector scanner at any security monitoring site

The possibility that a suitcase and its contents will become radioactive after passing through an airport X-ray scanner

Exposure to ultraviolet light for treating certain skin disease

Exposure to intense light and dermatologic chemicals for the treatment of acne

Eating food that has been sterilized by exposure to ionizing radiation

Other concerns of pregnant women in regard to radiation exposure include inadvertently being in a room when a radiograph was taken and being near a patient who has received external radiation therapy or who has been given a radionuclide for diagnostic or therapeutic purposes.

One must realize that families have grave concerns about having a child who has a birth defect, having a miscarriage, or having a child who has neurologic problems, mental retardation, or cancer following "radiation" exposures. Counselors must address these fears, even though many of them have no scientific basis. Discussion of all these matters in a compassionate and erudite manner can be of great benefit to concerned parents [66,81,82].

Clinical situations when a consultant is the primary prescriber of medications or therapies for diseases for which the obstetrician or perinatologist is not an expert

A proportion of obstetric and perinatology patients have medical problems that require special skills and training. Many of these special patients require medical care beyond the prenatal care and delivery services of an obstetrician or perinatologist. Many of these patients may need special medications, and it is important to review these medications with the medical consultant to make certain that the patient has been informed of any reproductive or developmental risks associated with these medications and whether alternative medications can be selected that do not reproductive or developmental risks. The patient's medical record should note the interaction with the consultant concerning the medications and that the information has been shared with the patient. Some perinatologists have been trained to care for diabetic pregnant patients or patients who have other complicated medical problems. It is advantageous for the perinatologist who is caring for pregnant patients who have complicated medical diseases to require that the patient's medical care be provided by the medical consultant. Diseases that necessitate the use of medications that may have reproductive or developmental risks include diabetes, malignancies, autoimmune disease, some infections, asthma or hyperactive airway disease, and any form of pulmonary or cardiac decompensation.

The perinatologist or obstetrician may not be an expert in many of these complicated medical diseases but can be very helpful to the medical consultant in selecting medications that are necessary for the patient that have either no increased risk or the least increased risk for reproductive or developmental problems.

How should a physician in respond to a citation that he or she is being sued for malpractice?

I have been a defense expert for many obstetricians, and on one occasion I was a plaintiff expert in an egregious case of malpractice that was settled before the trial began. I have the following suggestions for the defendants:

1. Immediately notify your insurance carrier, the hospital (if it is a hospital case), your partners, and appropriate members of your family.
2. Recognize that any competent attorney can study the medical aspects of the case and know more than you do at the time of the depositions and trial. Therefore, the three most important aspects of being a defendant are "preparation, preparation, and preparation."
3. Make certain that you have an excellent attorney and law firm. You have the right to request new counsel if you detect delays and incompetence.
4. Make certain that you have the best expert witnesses with absolutely no academic or ethical skeletons in their closet.
5. **Do not:**
   A. Go to the record room on the day you receive your citation and sign out the chart. You can look at your office records, but stay away from the record room until you have competent legal representation who will obtain the records in a proper manner.
   B. Call the plaintiff's attorney, even if you are friends or belong to the same organization or club.
   C. Call the plaintiff. Inform the patient that you are transferring her records to another physician. Your lawyer should supervise this correspondence.

   D. Contact other defendants or potential defendants in the case without advice from your attorney. If contact is made, your attorney should be present.
6. Be prepared for a lengthy process that is enervating, exhausting, and possibly anxiety-provoking. You will need the support of family, partners, attorney, and noninvolved colleagues.

What measures can scientists and physicians initiate to diminish the litigation epidemic?

Bendectin litigation is the prototype of nonmeritorious litigation, and the issues involved explain in part the epidemic of litigation brought before juries in this country. A lawsuit is filed because it may be won, regardless of whether it has merit [1,25,66,82]. A few changes could reduce the negligence litigation crisis and the excessive amount of nonmeritorious litigation in the United States.

The first suggestion is to eliminate the contingency-fee system for attorney compensation, a system that is practically nonexistent in the rest of the world. It is unlikely that this suggestion is going to be adopted for a long time in the United States, because the members of the law profession dominate the state and federal legislatures and have an undue influence on a significant proportion of the legislators [1,25].

The second suggestion is to put a cap on the size of the awards, especially on punitive damages. This suggestion has reduced litigation in some venues, but it will not solve the crisis.

The third suggestion is to eliminate the use of plaintiff and defense expert witnesses and rely on expert scientific panels that are "friends of the court." I discussed this matter many years ago [1]. I found out, however, that many of the plaintiff and defense attorneys want to use experts whom they select. Attorneys do not want a panel of court-assigned experts.

The fourth and most important suggestion is to have the loser pay the court costs. This measure would reduce dramatically the number of nonmeritorious lawsuits. It would discourage plaintiffs from filing nonmeritorious lawsuits and would encourage insurance companies to defend their clients rather than settle the nonmeritorious lawsuits, which is one of the large item costs in handling malpractice lawsuits. Assessing the court costs to the loser would change in the number of negligence lawsuits radically.

As physicians and scientists, we must recognize that the only area of litigation over which science and medicine can have legitimate control is in the performance of expert witnesses. Most nonmeritorious cases would not proceed if the attorneys could not find a physician or scientist who is willing to say that a nonmeritorious case has merit. Therefore, although we may be displeased with some attorneys and may blame them for the epidemic of litigation, the fact is that unscrupulous scientists and physicians have an important role in promoting nonmeritorious actions. Because we are not able to modernize the legal system, our best initiative is to alter drastically the activities of the irresponsible expert by raising the quality of expert-witness testimony [23,54,66,82]. We must strengthen the guidelines of universities and professional organizations in the United States to train and encourage scientists and physicians to perform as scholars and to monitor their contributions to the courts. If they do not provide competent and scholarly testimony, they should be criticized or expelled by their universities or their professional scientific and medical organizations.

Summary

Although some aspects of this discussion may seem to be critical of the legal profession, it is important to place this criticism into perspective. Physicians, as a group, tend to be hypercritical of the legal profession because of the escalation of malpractice litigation and malpractice insurance premiums. Recommendations from the medical community to modify the law to reduce the frequency of nonmeritorious litigation and the size of the awards have been minimally successful, primarily because lawyers dominate the legislatures. Furthermore, many attempts by physicians to change the law are naive. My suggestions in the past have urged the medical community to focus their attention on junk scientists and their junk science, because they are problems that emanate from the medical community, over which physicians should have some authority [1,23,25].

More importantly, we should respect the importance and accomplishments of the legal profession and admire its accomplishments, because it is the foundation of any thriving democracy. Without the law, we could never have rid ourselves of a sitting president or protect all rights bestowed on individuals in our Constitution. A very small percentage of attorneys exploiting the power of the law to their own advantage does not mean that the legal system must be replaced or eliminated. It is to everyone's advantage to have a functioning legal system with its benefits and risks. Remember that many nonmeritorious lawsuits could not proceed without the testimony of a junk scientist who appears before a judge and testifies that the case has merit. Many of these junk scientists are obstetricians and pediatricians as well as other members of the clinical and scientific community [49–51].

Will the situation improve? I cannot predict the future of malpractice litigation, but we are not doing our job by allowing irresponsible expert witnesses to participate in matters of litigation without being censured by their university or professional organizations [47,49–51].

References

[1] Brent RL. Medicolegal aspects of teratology. J Pediatr 1967;71:288–98.
[2] Fraser FC. Causes of congenital malformations in humans. J Chronic Dis 1959;10:97–110.

[3] Wilson JG. Factors involved in causing congenital malformations. Bull N Y Acad Med 1960; 16:145.

[4] Warkany J, Kalter H. Congenital malformations. N Engl J Med 1961;265:993, 1046.

[5] Karnofsky DA. Drugs as teratogens in animals and man. Ann Rev Pharmacol 1965;5: 447–72.

[6] Mellin GW. Drugs in the first trimester of pregnancy and fetal life of Homo sapiens. Am J Obst Gynecol 1964;90:1169–80.

[7] Wilson JG. Environment and birth defects. New York: Academic Press; 1973.

[8] Brent RL, Harris M. The prevention of embryonic fetal and perinatal disease; Bethesda (MD), US Govt. Publication DHEW Publ. NIH 76-853. 1975. p. 411.

[9] Beckman DA, Brent RL. Fetal effects of prescribed and self-administered drugs during the second and third trimester. In: Avery GB, Fletcher MA, MacDonald MG, editors. Neonatology: pathophysiology and treatment. 4th edition. Philadelphia: JB Lippincott Company; 1994. p. 197–206.

[10] Brent RL, Beckman DA. Prescribed drugs, therapeutic agents, and fetal teratogenesis. In: Reece EA, Hobbins JC, editors. Medicine of the fetus and mother. 2nd edition. Philadelphia: Lippincott-Raven Publishers; 1999. p. 289–313.

[11] Brent RL. Environmental causes of human congenital malformations: the pediatrician's role in dealing with these complex clinical problems caused by a multiplicity of environmental and genetic factors. Pediatrics 2004;113(4):957–68.

[12] Warkany J. Congenital malformation: notes and comments. Chicago: Year Book Medical Publishers; 1971.

[13] Warkany J. Congenital malformations in the past. J Chronic Dis 1959;10:84–95.

[14] Warkany J, Kalter H. Maternal impressions and congenital malformations. Plast Reconstr Surg 1962;30:628–37.

[15] Headley CJ. Records of the colony and plantation of New Haven from 1638 to 1649. Hartford (CT): Case Tiffany & Co; 1857.

[16] Landauer W. Hybridization between animals and man as a cause of congenital malformations. Extra Arch Anat Histol Embryol Normales et Exper 1961;14(Suppl):155–68.

[17] Sinkler appellant, v Kneale, 401 Pa., Appeal No. 124, January 1960, from order of the Court of Common Pleas of Chester County, March 1, 1959. No. 49, of Sinkler v Kneale, 1960; 267–78.

[18] Lejeune J, Turpin R, Gauteir M. Le mongolisme, maladie chromosomique (trisomie). Bull Acad Nat Med 1959;143:256–65.

[19] Patau K, Smith DW, Therman E, et al. Multiple congenital anomaly caused by an extra autosome. Lancet 1960;9:790–3.

[20] Makino S. Chromosomal studies in normal human subjects in 300 cases of congenital disorders. Int J Cytol 1964;9(1):13–31.

[21] Caroll v Skloff 159: In the Supreme Court of Pennsylvania, Eastern District No. 131, January 1, 1964. Appeal from the Judgment of the Court of Common Pleas No. 1 of Philadelphia County, March Term, 1963, No. 5407, sustaining appellees' preliminary objections and dismissing appellants' complaint, Entered October 25, 1963.

[22] Churchill J. Rights of the fetus to sue. Br Med J 1973;224.

[23] Brent RL. The irresponsible expert witness: a failure of biomedical graduate education and professional accountability. Pediatrics 1982;70:754–62.

[24] Physician Insurers Association of America. Available at: http://www.piaa.us/about_piaa/ what_is_piaa.htm.

[25] Brent RL. Litigation-produced pain, disease and suffering: an experience with congenital malformation lawsuits. Teratology 1977;16:1–14.

[26] Beckman DA, Fawcett LB, Brent RL. Developmental toxicity. In: Massaro EJ, editor. Handbook of human toxicology. New York: CRC Press; 1997. p. 1007–84.

[27] Brent RL. Non-genital malformations following exposure to progestational drugs: the final chapter of an erroneous allegation. Birth Defects, Part A 2005;73(11):906–18.

[28] Gal I, Kirman B, Stern J. Hormonal pregnancy tests and congenital malformations. Nature 1967;216:83.

[29] Janerich DT, Piper JM, Glebatis DM. Oral contraceptives and congenital limb-reduction defects. N Engl J Med 1974;291(14):697–700.

[30] Levy EP, Cohen A, Fraser FC. Hormone treatment during pregnancy and congenital heart. Lancet 1973;1:611.

[31] Heinonen OP, Sloane D, Monson RR, et al. Cardiovascular birth defects and antenatal exposure to female sex hormones. N Eng J Med 1977;296:67–70.

[32] Heinonen OP, Slone D, Shapiro S. Birth defects and drugs in pregnancy. Littleton (MA): Publishing Sciences Group Inc; 1977. p. 126–48.

[33] Nora JJ, Nora AH. Preliminary evidence for a possible association between oral contraceptives and birth defects. Teratology 1973;7:A24.

[34] Nora JJ, Nora AH. Birth defects and oral contraceptives. Lancet 1973;1:941–2.

[35] Nora JJ, Nora AH, Perinchief AG, et al. Congenital abnormalities and first-trimester exposure to progestogen/estrogen. Lancet 1976;1:313–4.

[36] Nora AH, Nora JJ. A syndrome of multiple congenital anomalies associated with teratogenic exposure. Arch Environ Health 1975;30:17–21.

[37] Nora JJ, Nora AH, Blu J, et al. Exogenous progestogen and estrogen implicated in birth defects. JAMA 1978;240:837–43.

[38] Brent RL. Kudos to the Food and Drug Administration: reversal of the package insert warning for birth defects for oral contraceptives. Teratology 1989;39(1):93–4.

[39] Food and Drug Administration. Progestational drug products for human use; requirements for labeling directed to the patient. Federal Register, Vol. 64, No. 70, Proposed Rules, Department of Health and Human Services (HHS), Public Health Service (PHS), Food and Drug Administration (FDA), 21 CFR Part 310, [Docket No. 99N-0188], 64 FR 17985, Date: Tuesday, April 13, 1999.

[40] Wilson JG, Brent RL. Are female sex hormones teratogenic? Am J Obstet Gynecol 1981; 141(5):567–80.

[41] Nocke W. Sind weibliche sexualsteroide teratogen? Ruckblick-Zwischenbilanz-Konsequenzen. Gynakologe 1978;11:119–41 [in German].

[42] Are sex steroids teratogenic? [editorial]. Lancet 1974;l:1489–90.

[43] Holmes LB. Teratogen update: bendectin. Teratology 1983;27(2):277–81.

[44] Brent RL. The bendectin saga: another American tragedy (Brent, '80). Teratology 1983;27: 283–6.

[45] Brent RL. Bendectin and interventricular septal defects [editorial]. Teratology 1985;32: 317–8.

[46] Brent RL. Teratogen update: bendectin [editorial comments]. Teratology 1985;31:429–30.

[47] Lasagna L, Shulman SR. Bendectin and the language of causation. In: Foster KR, Bernsyein DE, Huber PW, editors. Phantom risk: scientific interference and the law. Cambridge (MA): MIT Press; 1993. p. 101–22.

[48] Brent RL. Commentary: bringing scholarship to the courtroom: the Daubert decision and its impact on the Teratology Society. Teratology 1995;52:247–51.

[49] Brent RL. Bendectin: review of the medical literature of a comprehensively studied human non-teratogen and the most prevalent tortogen-litigen. Reprod Toxicol 1995;9(4): 337–49.

[50] Brent RL. Review of the scientific literature pertaining to the reproductive toxicity of bendectin. In: Faigman DL, Kaye DH, Saks MJ, et al, editors. Modern scientific evidence: the law and science of expert testimony. vol. 2. St. Paul (MN): West Publishing Group; 1997. p. 373–93.

[51] Brent RL. Medical, social and legal implications of treating nausea and vomiting of pregnancy. Am J Obstet Gynecol 2002,186(5):S262–6.

[52] Kutcher JS, Engle A, Firth J, et al. Bendectin and birth defects. II: ecological analyses. Birth Defects Res A Clin Mol Teratol 2003;67(2):88–97.

[53] Brent RL. Commentary on bendectin and birth defects: hopefully, the final chapter. Birth Defects Res A Clin Mol Teratol 2003;67(2):79–87.

[54] Skolnick A. Key witness against morning sickness drug faces scientific fraud charges. JAMA 1990;283:1466–9.

[55] Hanson JW, Smith DW. The fetal hydantoin syndrome. Teratology 1975;11(2):20A.

[56] OMIM, Online Mendelian inheritance in man. Available at: http://www.ncbi.nlm.nih.gov/entrez/query.fcgi?db=OMIM. Accessed October 12, 2006.

[57] Friedman JM, Polifka JE. TERIS. The teratogen information system. Seattle (WA): University of Washington; 1999.

[58] Scialli AR, Lione A, Padget GKB, editors. Reproductive effects of chemical, physical and biologic agents: Reprotox. Baltimore (MD): The Johns Hopkins University Press; 1995.

[59] Sever JL, Brent RL, editors. Teratogen update: environmentally induced birth defect risks. New York: Alan R. Liss; 1986. p. 1–248.

[60] Shepard TH. Catalogue of teratogenic agents. 8th edition. Baltimore (MD): The Johns Hopkins University Press; 1995.

[61] Schardein JL. Chemically induced birth defects. 3rd edition. New York: Marcel Dekker, Inc.; 2000.

[62] Briggs GG, Freeman RK, Yaffe SJ. Drugs in pregnancy and lactation. 3rd edition. Baltimore (MD): Williams and Wilkins; 1990. p. 502–8.

[63] Brent RL. Utilization of developmental basic science principles in the evaluation of reproductive risks from pre- and postconception environmental radiation exposures. Presented at the thirty-third annual meeting of the National Council on Radiation Protection and Measurements. The Effects of Pre- and Postconception Exposure to Radiation. Arlington (VA), April 2–3, 1997. Teratology 1999;59:182–204.

[64] Brent RL, Holmes LB. Clinical and basic science lessons from the thalidomide tragedy: what have we learned about the causes of limb defects? Teratology 1988;38:241–51.

[65] Brent RL. Methods of evaluating the alleged teratogenicity of environmental agents. In: Sever JL, Brent RL, editors. Teratogen update: environmentally induced birth defect risks. New York: Alan R. Liss; 1986. p. 199–201.

[66] Brent RL. Improving the quality of expert witness testimony. Pediatrics 1988;82:511–3.

[67] Brent RL, Koren G, Scialli A, et al. Report on the safety of bendectin/Diclectin for use in the management of nausea and vomiting of pregnancy. Ottawa, Canada: Health Protection Branch; 1989.

[68] Food and Drug Administration. Department of Health and Human Services. Determination that bendectin was not withdrawn from sale for reasons of safety or effectiveness. Docket nos. 92F and 97)-G437. 64 Federal Register 43190–1; 1999.

[69] Brent RL, Beckman DA. Angiotensin converting enzyme inhibitors: an embryopathic class of drugs with unique properties: information for clinical teratology counselors. Teratology 1991;43:543–6.

[70] Barr M. Teratogen update: angiotensin converting enzyme inhibitors. Teratology 1994;50: 399–409.

[71] Al-Shabanah OA, Al-Harbi MM, AlGharably NMA, et al. The effect of maternal administration of captopril on fetal development in the rat. Res Commun Chem Pathol Pharmacol 1994;73:221–30.

[72] Alwan S, Polifka J, Friedman JM. Angiotensin II receptor antagonist treatment during pregnancy. Birth Defects Res A Clin Mol Teratol 2005;73:123–30.

[73] Cooper WO, Hernandez-Diaz S, Arbogast PG, et al. Major congenital malformations after first-trimester exposure to ACE inhibitors. New Engl J Med 2006;354:2443–51.

[74] Kallen B, Otterblad Olausson P. Antidepressant drugs during pregnancy and infant congenital heart defect. Reprod Toxicol 2006;21:221–2.

[75] Diav-Citrin O, Shechtman S, Weinbaum D, et al. Paroxetine and fluoxetine in pregnancy: a multicenter, prospective, controlled study. Reprod Toxicol 2005;20(3):459.

[76] Kulin NA, Pastuszak A, Sage SR, et al. Pregnancy outcome following maternal use of the new selective serotonin reuptake inhibitors. A prospective controlled multicenter study. JAMA 1998;279(8):609–10.

[77] Rosa F. New medical entities widely used in fertile women: postmarketing surveillance priorities. Reprod Toxicol 1995;9(6):583.

[78] Brent RL, Jones CG, Roessler GS. Internet communications with the public: a new powerful health physics society tool. Presented at the eleventh International Congress of the International Radiation Protection Association. Madrid (Spain), May 23–28, 2004. Available at: http://www.irpa11.com. Accessed June 6, 2004.

[79] Jones CG, Roessler GS, Brent RL. Effective radiological communications with the public. Strahlenschutz Praxis 2004;4:23–7.

[80] Brent RL. Counseling patients exposed to ionizing radiation during pregnancy. Rev Panam Salud Publica 2006;20:198–205.

[81] Brent RL. Microwaves and ultrasound. In: Queenan JT, Hobbins JC, Spong CY, editors. Protocols high-risk pregnancy: a contemporary OB/GYN. 4th edition. Malden (MA): Blackwell Publishing; 2005. p. 39–44.

[82] Brent RL. Malpractice experience and issues. In: Medical-legal issues in pediatrics, report of the eighteenth Ross roundtable on critical approaches to common pediatric problems in collaboration with the Ambulatory Pediatric Association. Columbus (OH): Ross Laboratories; 1987. p. 20–5.

ELSEVIER
SAUNDERS

CLINICS IN
PERINATOLOGY

Clin Perinatol 34 (2007) 263–273

Congenital Disabilities and the Law

Robert Roth, BA, LLB

Sommers & Roth, Professional Corporation, 268 Avenue Road,
Toronto, Ontario M4V 2G7, Canada

Congenital disabilities and the law involves medical negligence in failing to test or interpret tests to provide parents with information to enable them to choose to terminate a pregnancy. No other area of civil negligence law gives rise to the kind of emotional, philosophic, theologic, and passionate analysis as the claims that have been designated, as "wrongful conception," "wrongful birth," and "wrongful life." The fact that most reported court decisions use quotation marks around these terms emphasizes a discomfort with the pejorative nature of the terms and the emotive labeling that has developed in the law in this area.

The claims

"Wrongful conception"

The claim for "wrongful conception" does not necessarily arise as the result of a child born with a congenital disability. This claim may involve, for example, a failed vasectomy or tubal ligation that was sought by parents who determined that, as a matter of family planning, they did not wish to bear more children. The claim is sometimes referred to as "wrongful pregnancy." The complaint arises before conception takes place. Often a healthy child is born, but birth was unplanned. Courts have recognized the validity of the parents' claim in this regard, although there is disagreement on the proper measure of damages.

In England, the courts have allowed damages for all child-rearing costs arising from failed sterilization procedures [1]. In the United States, a few state courts have permitted total recovery of all damages flowing proximately from a physician's negligence [2]. This followed earlier decisions refusing damages for a healthy but unplanned child [3].

E-mail address: rroth@sommersandroth.com

0095-5108/07/$ - see front matter © 2007 Elsevier Inc. All rights reserved.
doi:10.1016/j.clp.2007.03.004
perinatology.theclinics.com

Another approach to damages in "wrongful conception" cases is the "off-setting benefits" approach, whereby the "benefits for the unplanned child may be weighed against the elements of the claimed damages" [4]. Many United States courts apply a "limited damages" approach and allow damages for the pain and suffering associated with the labor and delivery and the costs of a second sterilization procedure [5]. The rationale for the "limited damages" approach parallels the rationale in certain jurisdictions that refuse to recognize a child's claim for "wrongful life" (eg, the sanctity of life, the protection of the mental and emotional health of the child, or any damages that are too speculative or remote). The Supreme Court of Illinois, using an analysis commonly seen in this area of law, stated:

> One can, of course, in mechanical logic reach a different conclusion, but only on the ground that human life and the state of parenthood are compensable losses. In a proper hierarchy of values, the benefit of life should not be outweighed by the cost of supporting it. Respect for life and the rights proceeding from it are at the heart of our legal system and broader still, our civilization [6].

In Ontario, in an early case involving "wrongful conception", the court expressed its opinion as follows:

> Personally, I find this approach to a matter of this kind which deals with human life, the happiness of the child, the effect upon its thinking, upon its mind when it realizes that there has been a case of this kind, that it is an unwanted mistake, and that its rearing is being paid for by someone other than its parents, is just simply grotesque [7].

In an enlightened subsequent judgment in Ontario [8], the court recognized that there is no rule of public policy requiring people to have children or preventing them from determining the number of children they choose to have. It is a recognized community norm to allow parents the right to plan and limit the size of their families. The court stated that the time has long passed when a court is free to dismiss such a claim as "grotesque." Balancing the sentiment that favors sensible family planning with that which regards children as beneficial, the court left open the possibility that, in an action brought by parents seeking a sterilization procedure to avoid the imposition of an unreasonable financial burden on their family (or to protect a mother's health where she becomes ill, thus impairing her ability to care for a child), damages on a different scale could be considered.

Wrongful birth

The claim of "wrongful birth" is advanced by the parents of a child born with genetic defects wherein a physician or technician, for example, failed to order, carry out, or interpret appropriate tests during the pregnancy that would have disclosed the presence of the defect, allowing the physician or technician to inform the parents of its presence. The claim is predicated on the denial of appropriate information to the parents, due to negligence, to entitle the parents to make an informed decision whether to terminate the pregnancy. The claim is brought by such parents on their own behalf and is based on negligent interference with the mother's lawful right to choose whether or not to terminate the pregnancy. The negligence may arise, for instance, where a physician fails to warn a pregnant woman of the increased risk of damage to her fetus from exposure to German measles in the first trimester It may also entail a failure to advise or recommend to a pregnant woman the availability of amniocentesis, it may involve negligent genetic counseling for a number of known conditions, or it may involve negligent misinterpretation of an ultrasound disclosing the presence of a neural tube defect.

Most Anglo-American courts have recognized the validity of a cause of action for "wrongful conception" and "wrongful birth" [9]. The controversy continues with respect to the range of damages that may be awarded. This cause of action was not always recognized and is not universally accepted.

In 1967, the New Jersey Court, in Gleitman v Cosgrove [10], considered a claim by parents regarding a child who was born deaf, mute, and nearly blind as a result of being exposed to rubella in utero. The physician had advised the mother that there was no risk that such exposure would harm the fetus. The mother testified that had she been given proper advice, she would have terminated the pregnancy. In dismissing the child's claim, the court decided that such a claim "did not give rise to damages cognizable at law." The court expressed an oft repeated concern with regard to a child's claim; that is, the impossibility of measuring the child's damages on traditional tort principles, which would require a comparison of the child's life with defects against non-existence [10].

The court also rejected the parents' claim for "wrongful birth" because "the right of their child to live is greater than, and precludes, their right not to endure emotional and financial injury" [10]. The court stressed the difficulty of weighing the emotional and financial burdens to the parents against the "immeasurable and complex human benefits of motherhood and fatherhood" [10].

Gleitman was decided before the American Supreme Court's decision in Roe v. Wade [11], which had a major impact on this area of law. That decision, which determined that women have a constitutional right to an abortion during the first trimester of pregnancy, resulted in courts being more favorably responsive to a parent's "wrongful birth" claim. Indeed, in New Jersey, despite its decision in Gleitman, that state's court revisited the "wrongful birth" claim 12 years later and reversed its earlier ruling, noting that "to deny [parents] redress for their injuries merely because damages cannot be measured with precise exactitude would constitute a perversion of the fundamental principles of natural justice" [12].

In 1985, the Supreme Court of Idaho said:

> Clearly the arguments once found persuasive in denying the wrongful birth actions have lost their potency. Furthermore, we note at least two policy considerations which have been advanced in favor of recognizing the cause of action. The first is based upon the expanding ability of medicine to predict and detect birth defects before conception or birth. Imposing liability on individual physicians vindicates the societal interest in reducing the incidence of genetic defects. The other consideration flows from general tort principles. A physician whose negligence has deprived a woman of the opportunity to make an informed decision whether her fetus should be aborted should be required to compensate her for the damage proximately caused. 'Any other ruling would in effect immunize from liability those in the medical field providing inadequate guidance to persons who would choose to exercise their constitutional right to abort fetuses which, if born, would suffer from genetic defects' [13].

Usually, the parents' damage claims are primarily to recover the extraordinary costs of providing for their disabled child's special needs. There remains the controversial and unresolved question of whether the parents' claim to recover the extraordinary expenses of medical care, attendant care, equipment, physiotherapy, transportation, housing, etc., required for their child's lifelong needs arising from the condition ends when the child reaches the age of majority or continues so long as the parent assumes responsibility for the child's care needs.

Despite the general trend of the courts in North America and England to accept the parents' claim as a valid cause of action, 11 states have, by legislation or court decisions, prohibited the parents' claims [14]; this is a minority view but is one that underlines the continuing debate and volatile nature of this area of law.

"Wrongful life"—to be or not to be

The claim that has generated and continues to generate the most emotive resistance in the courts is the child's claim. In this article, I emphasize the minority view that recognizes this claim. The philosophical question raised by this claim is best encapsulated in Hamlet's soliloquy:

> To be or not to be; that is the question
>
> Whether 'tis nobler to the mind to suffer
>
> The slings and arrows of outrageous fortune
>
> Or to take arms against a sea of troubles
>
> And by opposing, end them.

An early decision by the Court of Appeal of New York in 1978 reflects the reluctance of the court to accept the claim by the child:

Whether it is better never to have been born at all than to have been born with even gross deficiencies is a mystery more properly to be left to the philosophers and the theologians. Surely, the law can assert no competence to resolve the issue, particularly in view of the very nearly uniform high value which the law and mankind has placed on human life rather than its absence [15].

In other words, life itself cannot be an injury.

The court then adopted a second basis for resisting the child's claim, namely that "a cause of action brought on behalf of an infant seeking recovery for wrongful life demands a calculation of damages dependent upon a comparison between the Hobson's choice of life in an impaired state and non-existence. This comparison, the law is not equipped to make" [15].

In 1990, the Supreme Judicial Court of Massachusetts criticized the use of the terms "wrongful conception," "wrongful birth," and "wrongful life," with the observation that the terms were confusing and misleading. That court pointed out that the "wrongfulness" lies not in the life, the birth, the conception, or the pregnancy but is in the negligence of the physician. The court went on to state that "the harm is not the birth itself, but the effect of the defendant's negligence on the parents' physical, emotional and financial well-being resulting from the denial to the parents of their right to decide whether to bear a child with a genetic or other defect" [16].

Most courts have refused to recognize a child's right to assert a claim for damages on his own behalf because of alleged inability to compute damages based on a measurement of the difference between life in an impaired condition and nonexistence and a refusal to recognize a lawful duty of a physician to a fetus to end its life.

Three American state courts have given recognition to the child's claim [17]. In England and Canada, no court has recognized the claim for the child [18]. The issue has been considered elsewhere. In France, the Cour de Cassation (Supreme Court) gave recognition to a child's claim, only to be followed by legislation prohibiting such claims [19]. In Israel, the Supreme Court has recognized the child's right to assert a claim and recover damages [20]. Tort law has been described as a living tree with new torts being recognized as society evolves. The unwillingness of courts to assess damages for a child's claim, professing the inability to monetarily restore the child to the condition he would have been in but for the negligence (ie, the genetic condition was not brought about in consequence of a negligent act; an impaired life was) leading to a refusal to recognize the cause of action, is a narrow and restrictive application of tort law. In a leading textbook on tort law, Prosser and Keeton describe tort law's goal as follows:

> The law of torts…is concerned with the allocation of losses arising out of human activities…of persons living in a common society…The purpose of the law of torts is to adjust these losses, and to afford compensation for injuries sustained by one person as a result of the conduct of another [21].

The foremost decision upholding the child's entitlement to a claim is Curlender v Bio-Science Laboratories [22], wherein the California Court of Appeal set forth the following basis for accepting the claim:

> Public Policy, as perceived by most courts, has been used as the basis for denying recovery; in some fashion, a deeply held belief in the sanctity of life has compelled some courts to deny recovery to those among us who have been born with serious impairment…
>
> We have alluded to the monumental implications of Roe v. Wade, one of which is the present legality of, and availability of, eugenic abortion, in the proper case. Another factor of substantial proportions in 'wrongful life' litigation is the dramatic increase, in the last few decades of the medical knowledge and skill needed to avoid genetic disaster…
>
> We have no difficulty in asserting and finding the existence of a duty owed by medical laboratories engaged in genetic testing to parents and their as yet unborn children to use ordinary care in administration of available tests for the purpose of providing information concerning potential genetic defects in the unborn…
>
> The real crux of the problem is whether the breach of duty was the proximate cause of an injury cognizable at law. The injury, of course, is not the particular defect with which a plaintiff is afflicted – considered in the abstract – but it is the birth of the plaintiff with such defect…
>
> The circumstance that the birth and injury have come hand in hand has caused other courts to deal with the problem by barring recovery. The reality of the 'wrongful life' concept is that such a plaintiff both exists and suffers due to the negligence of others. It is neither necessary nor just to retreat into meditation on the mysteries of life. We need not be concerned with the fact that had the defendants not been negligent, the plaintiff might not have come into existence at all. The certainty of genetic impairment is no longer a mystery. In addition, a reverent appreciation of life compels recognition that the plaintiff, however impaired she may be, has come into existence as a living person with certain rights…
>
> The 'wrongful life' cause of action with which we are concerned is based upon negligently caused failure by someone under a duty to do so to inform the prospective parents of facts needed by them to make a conscious choice *not* to become parents.

Subsequently, the Supreme Court of California reversed the Appellate Court's decision in Curlender, insofar as that court would have allowed the child to recover general damages for pain and suffering, but upheld the child's right to maintain a claim for his extraordinary expenses:

> Unlike the child's claim for general damages, the damages here are both certain and readily measurable. Furthermore, in many instances these expenses will be vital not only to the child's well-being, but to his or her very survival...Although the parents and child cannot, of course, both recover for the same medical expenses, we believe it would be illogical and anomalous to permit only parents, and not the child, to recover for the cost of the child's own medical care [23].

The recognition of that child's entitlement, and the rationale in respect thereof, bears comparison to the stark general refusal to allow that child's right to assert a claim to maintain himself given the impairments he will have throughout life.

The evolution of the law of torts in a somewhat comparable situation led to the acceptance of the right of a child, injured *in utero* by someone's negligence, to assert a claim for damages for those injuries, after he/she is born. In a 1933 decision, the first in Canada to decide the right of a child who sustains prenatal injury due to another's negligence, to maintain an action, the Supreme Court of Canada said:

> If a child after birth has no right of action for prenatal injuries, we have a wrong inflicted for which there is no remedy, for, although the father may be entitled to compensation for the loss he has incurred and the mother for what she has suffered, yet there is a residuum of injury for which compensation cannot be had save at the suit of the child. If a right of action be denied to the child, it will be compelled, without any fault on its part, to go through life carrying the seal of another's fault and bearing a very heavy burden of infirmity and inconvenience without any compensation therefore. To my mind, it is but natural justice that a child, if born alive and viable, should be allowed to maintain an action in the courts for injuries wrongfully committed upon its person while in the womb of its mother [24].

Considering the fact that most courts in North America have recognized as valid a claim by the parents of a child disabled by a negligently undetected genetic condition, which negligence prevented them from making the informed choice to terminate the pregnancy, and will award the parents damages, inter alia, for the extraordinary costs of providing necessary care for their child (at least until the child reaches the age of majority), is there not a residuum of injury to the child who has a lifetime need for extraordinary care? Is this anomalous situation, which awards damages to enable parents to provide for the extraordinary care needs of the child but denies damages to the child who directly has the need for extraordinary care, an acceptable position?

Most courts that refuse to recognize the child's claim for "wrongful life" do so on a perceived public policy that favors the sanctity of life, even in an impaired condition, over an alternative state of nonexistence. In other situations, the courts have recognized that the sanctity of life may not be an absolute value and that, in some circumstances, "non-life" may indeed be preferable to an "impaired life." In Re Quinlan [25], the court permitted parents, as guardians of a 22-year-old woman in a persistent vegetative state, to withdraw life support and thereby terminate her life. The court recognized that the value of continuing that life could be outweighed by ending that life.

In a California case involving the court's consideration of a patient's wish to remove a nasogastric feeding tube that had been inserted against her will and without her consent by physicians to keep her alive via involuntary forced feeding [26], the court decided that a patient who was mentally competent and understood the risks had a right to refuse treatment. The court went on to say that the State's interest in preserving life did not outweigh a patient's right to refuse treatment.

In Canada, the Ontario Court of Appeal considered the case of a Jehovah's Witness who was severely injured in an automobile accident and taken unconscious to a hospital. A nurse found a card in the patient's purse identifying herself as a Jehovah's Witness and requesting, on the basis of her religious beliefs, that she not be given a blood transfusion under any circumstances. The physician attending believed a blood transfusion was necessary to preserve the patient's life and health and gave the patient a blood transfusion in the belief that it was his professional responsibility to do so. Upon her recovery, the patient sued the physician, alleging the blood transfusion constituted negligence and assault and battery. The plaintiff's claim succeeded. The court stated [27]:

> The State's interest in preserving the life or health of a competent patient must generally give way to a patient's stronger interest in directing the course of her own life. As indicated earlier, there is no law prohibiting a patient from declining necessary treatment or prohibiting a doctor from honoring the patient's decision. To the extent that the law reflects the State's interest, it supports the right of individuals to make their own decisions.

This type of reasoning underlines the general acceptance of a parent's claim for damages for being denied the right to make an informed choice whether or not to terminate a pregnancy to avoid giving birth to a child who has a genetically caused impairment. Why does it not apply equally to the child's right? In part because courts have refused to acknowledge a duty owed to a fetus by a physician to end its life.

A parent faced with information that the child will be born with significant impairment who chooses to terminate the pregnancy does so for personal reasons of being unwilling to accept the burden of raising a handicapped child. Additionally, most parents would do so out of love and concern for the child, not wishing him/her to endure a life of hardship and deprivation. In our society, parents inevitably and regularly make decisions that affect the well-being of their children on behalf of those children.

In a review conducted at a hospital with a significant obstetrical unit, it was determined that greater than 90% of women elected to terminate their pregnancy when advised that the presence of a neural tube defect had been identified by ultrasound or maternal serum screening. Standards of practice require the physician to discuss such a finding with the pregnant woman and to discuss the options of termination or continuation of the pregnancy in the circumstances. Thus, some courts' insistence that life is sacred under any circumstance and that nonexistence can never be preferable to impaired existence may not be a value judgment shared by society at large. Indeed, the medical profession itself, in the exercise of its professional responsibility, acts in a manner that is in opposition to many courts' and legislatures' expressed position that life itself cannot be "wrongful" and cannot itself constitute an injury and to the belief that even an impaired life is preferable to nonlife.

In most hospitals in North America, after the birth of a child who has significant medical impairments, physicians discuss the condition and prognosis with the parents, and, depending on the parents' decision after that informed consent discussion, Do Not Resuscitate Orders may be written with respect to the child such that life-saving or life-preserving measures will not be provided.

Society accepts that parents are the primary proxy decision-makers for their children. As such, they have wide discretion to make decisions concerning the child's welfare. If a parent decided, after the birth of a disabled child, that the child's life would be beset, for example, by intractable pain or no possibility of human interaction or endeavor, the parent could make the choice to end the child's life with a Do Not Resuscitate Order. The medical profession ethically supports the parents' right to decide on behalf of their live-born child in this regard. The courts have lagged behind in recognizing a parent's right to decide on behalf of their unborn child.

The claim for "wrongful life" is based on the premise that, as the proxy decision maker for the fetus, parents are entitled to nonnegligent testing and advice from the physician not only to make an informed choice on their own behalf to terminate a pregnancy but also to make an informed choice on behalf of the fetus to terminate the pregnancy. The claim was clearly elucidated by the Supreme Court of New Jersey in 1984 [28]:

> The infant plaintiff's injury need not be defined as being born defective or require that non-existence be preferred to existence. Rather, his injury consists of the consequences of the deprivation of his parents' right to determine on his behalf whether he should have been born. What then is at issue as the basis for a cause of action is *not* the postulate that non-life is preferable to life, but only whether parents – for themselves and their child as a family – were deprived of the opportunity to make the fateful decision and enact their preference of one over the other...The child's complaint is predicated on the failure of the doctor to provide his parents with the ability to make informed choices on his behalf.

The controversy in this area of law reflects the controversy of the "right to life" movement in North America. The recent public and political furor that surrounded the decision to end the life of Theresa Schiavo by withdrawing life-prolonging use of a feeding tube emphasizes that passions and bitter conflicts continue. Clearly, society has an interest in protecting and promoting life. Society also has an interest in protecting and promoting the constitutional right to abortion and the "allocation of losses arising out of human activities." In a case decided in the Supreme Court of Pennsylvania, that court held [29]:

> We are not confronted here simply with the birth of an unwanted but healthy child. Before us, unfortunately, is a living and breathing, but incurably diseased, deformed, and suffering human being who never had a chance to be born healthy and who will be in need of extraordinary medical and other special care for the rest of her days. Any argument that this life of suffering is not the natural and probable consequence of (the physician's) misconduct is rank sophistry. To permit such a wrong to go unredressed would provide no deterrent to professional irresponsibility and be neither just nor compatible with this commonwealth's principles of tort liability.

The argument in favor of a child's claim is not based on a preference of nonexistence over existence. The injured child does not claim damages for the causing of life or the prevention of nonlife. Rather, the claim is with respect to a negligent act that results in a defective life. As stated by the court in Curlender, "The reality of the 'wrongful life' concept is that such plaintiff both exists and suffers due to the negligence of others" [30].

Summary

The majority of courts in North America have recognized the validity of claims for "wrongful conception" and "wrongful birth." The majority of the same courts have refused to accept claims brought by an injured child for "wrongful life." The evolution of the child's claim has stalled but is not at an end. Public policy, which has been described as a slippery slope, continues to be used by the courts to justify a refusal to recognize this claim. Future change in the perception of the applicable public policy will affect developments in this controversial area of law.

References

[1] Emeh v Kensington and Chelsea and Westminster Health Authority, [1984] 3 All E.R. 1044 (C.A.) and Thake v Maurice, [1984] 2 All E.R. 513, aff'd (1986) 1 All E.R. 497 (C.A.).
[2] Custodio v Bauer, 251 Cal. App. 2d 303 (1967); Stills v Gratton, 55 Cal. App 3d 698(1976).
[3] Shaheen v Knight, 6 Lycoming R.19; 11 L.D. & C 2d 41 (1957); Christensen v Thornby, 192 Minn. 123, 255 N.W. 620(1934).

[4] Troppi v Scarf, 187 N.W. 2d 511 (Mich. C.A. 1971); Kealey v Berezowski (1996), 136 D.L.R. (4th) 708; Ochs v Borrelli 187 Conn. 253; 445 A.2d 883 (Conn. Sup. Ct. 1982) Burke v Rivo, 406 Mass. 764, 551 N.E. 2d 1(1990).

[5] Wilczynski v Godman, 73 Ill. App. 3d 51; 391 N.E.2d 479 (1979); Mason v Western Pennsylvania Hospital; 453 A. 2d 974 (Pa. Supr. 1982); Wilber v Kerr, 275 Ark. 239, 628 S.W. 2d 568 (Ark. 1982); McKernan v Assheim, 102 Wash. 2d 411; 687 P. 2d 850(1984).

[6] Cokrum v Baumgartner, 95 Ill. 2d 193 at 203; 447 N.E. 2d 385 (1983).

[7] Doiron v Orr (1978), 20 O.R. (2d) 71 (Ont. H.C.) at 74.

[8] Kealey v Berezowski supra note 4.

[9] Blake v Cruz, 108 Idaho 253; 698 P.2d 315 (1984); Berman v Allen, 80 N.J. 421(1979); Schloss v. Miriam Hospital, [1999] WL 41875 (R.I. Superior Court); Garrison v Medical Centre of Delaware, 581 A.2d 288 (1989); Siemieniec v Lutheran General Hospital, 117 Ill. 2d 230 (1987); Smith v Cote, 128 N.H. 231; 513 A.2d 341 (1986); Becker v Schwartz, 386 N.E. 2d 807 (1978); Emeh v Kensington (1984), 3 All E.R. 1044 (C.A.); Thake v Maurice [1984], 2 All. E.R 513; aff'd 1 All E.R. 497 (C.A.).

[10] Gleitman v Cosgrove, 227 A.2d 689, 692, 693 (N.J. 1967).

[11] Roe v Wade, 410 U.S. 113 (1973); see also R. v Morgentaler [1988] 1 S.C.R. 30.

[12] Berman, supra note 9 at 15.

[13] Blake v Cruz, supra note 9 at 319.

[14] Idaho Code §5-334 (Michie 2000); Ind. Code § 34-12-1-1 (Michie 1989); Minnesota Stat. § 145, 424 (2000) Mo. Rev. Stat. § 188-130 (1) (1999) N.D. Cent. Code § 32-03-43 (2000) 42; Pa. Cons. Stat. § 8305(2000); S.D. Codified Laws § 21-55-1 (2000); Utah Code Ann. § 78-11-24 (2000); Wilbur v. Kerr, 628 S.W. 2d 568 (1982); Atlanta Obstetrics and Gynecology Group v Abelson, 398 S.E.2d 557 (Ga. 1990); Schork v Huber, 648 S.W. 2d 861 (Ky. 1983); Taylor v Kurapati, 600 N.W.2d 670 (Mich. Ct. App. 1999); Azzolino v Dingfelder, 337 S.E.2d 528 (N.C. 1985); Morris v Sanchez, 746 P.2d 184 (Okla. 1987).

[15] Becker v Schwartz, 386 N.E. 2d 807 at 812 (N.Y.C.A. 1978).

[16] Viccaro v Milunsky, 551 N.E. 2d 8 (Mass. 1990) at 10.

[17] Curlender v Bio-Sci Labs, 165 Cal. Rptr. 477 (Cal. C.A. 1980); Turpin v Sortini, 643 P. 2d 954 (Cal. Ct. App. 1982); Harbeson v Parke-Davis, 656 P.2d 483 (Wash. 1983); Procanik v Cillo, 478 A. 2d 755 (N.J. 1984).

[18] McKay v Essex Health Authority [1982], 2 All. E.R. 771 (C.A.); Lacroix v. Dominique, [2001] 202 D.L.R. (4th) 121 (Man. C.A.); Paxton v Ramji, [2006] O.J. No. 1179 (2006).

[19] Re Perruche—Cour de Cassation (Supreme Court of France), November 17, 2000, Arret/Conclusions/Rapport.

[20] Zeitzoff et al. v Katz, et al. (1986) 40 (2) PD 85 Supreme Court of Israel (translated into English by Dr. Zive Weil, " Wrongful Life: An Israeli Case. Transcript of proceedings of the Supreme Court Sitting as the Court of Appeals" (1990) 9 Med & Law at 865.).

[21] W Page Keeton, et al. Prosser and Keeton on Torts 5th ed. (St. Paul Minn: West Publishing Com1984) at 6.

[22] Curlender v Bio-Science Laboratories, 106 Cal. App. 3d 811 (1980) at 486–87.

[23] Turpin, supra note 21 at 965.

[24] Montreal Tramways v Leveille (1933), 4 D.L.R. 337 at 345 (S.C.C.).

[25] Re Quinlan, 355 A 2d 647 (1970).

[26] Bouvia v Superior Court, 225 Cal. Rptr. 297 (Cal. Ct. of Appeal. 1986).

[27] Malette v Shulman (1990), 72 O.R. (2d) 417 at 429.

[28] Procancik, supra note 21 at 769.

[29] Speck v Finegold, 497 Pa 77; 439 A.2d 110 (1981) at 118.

[30] Curlender, supra note 21 at 488.1.

ELSEVIER
SAUNDERS

CLINICS IN
PERINATOLOGY

Clin Perinatol 34 (2007) 275–285

Informed Consent

Laurence B. McCullough, PhD[a],*, Frank A. Chervenak, MD[b]

[a]Center for Medical Ethics and Health Policy, Baylor College of Medicine,
One Baylor Plaza, Houston, TX 77030, USA
[b]Department of Obstetrics and Gynecology, Weill Medical College of Cornell University,
525 East 68th Street–J130, New York, NY, USA

Informed consent is an essential component of the practice of perinatal medicine because, as a process of communication and decision making, it should shape the relationship between the physician and pregnant woman and between the physician and the parents of a newborn child. This important matter is often trivialized by physicians when they relegate to the most junior member of the team who instructed to "consent" the patient. This article provides an antidote to this unprofessional attitude and practice by providing an account of the physician's obligations in the informed consent process in terms of ethics and law. The law has deeply shaped the informed consent process, but ethics has as well in ways that are clinically significant for the practice of perinatal medicine.

Ethics, medical ethics, and law

Ethics has been understood in diverse global intellectual traditions for centuries to be the disciplined study of morality. Morality concerns our beliefs and attitudes concerning what sort of people we should become and how we should act toward each other. Medical morality concerns the policies and practices of physicians and health care organizations and the attitudes and behaviors of leaders of health care organizations. Medical ethics is the disciplined study of morality in medicine. The basic assumption of ethics generally and medical ethics specifically is that current morality is in need of critical scrutiny and continuous improvement. In medicine, the improvement of medical ethics is essential for improving the quality of patient care and protecting research subjects [1].

---

* Corresponding author.
E-mail address: mccullou@bcm.edu (L.B. McCullough).

0095-5108/07/$ - see front matter © 2007 Elsevier Inc. All rights reserved.
doi:10.1016/j.clp.2007.03.005

The improvement of medical morality specifically is accomplished in medical ethics by asking, and providing argued responses to, two basic questions. First, what sort of professionals ought physicians to become? This question concerns the virtues that physicians should cultivate, the vices that they should avoid, and the parallel kinds of organizational culture that physician leaders should cultivate or avoid [1]. Second, how should physicians act toward their patients, toward each other, toward health care organizations, and toward society generally? This question concerns the ethical principles that should guide the decisions and behaviors of individuals and that should guide the policies and practices of organizations [1,2].

Medical ethics is a tool of social control, the responsibility for which society has delegated to the medical profession. By contrast, law is a tool of social control created, administered, and enforced by state power. In the United States and other democracies, the ethical authority of law (ie, what commands our compliance with it) is the consent of the governed to the institutions of self-government. American law has four components: (1) statutory law, which is created by legislatures and enforced by courts and law enforcement authorities; (2) common law, which is written by judges, compliance to which is a function of the intellectual and political authority of the reasoning set forth by trial court, appellate, and supreme court justices in state and federal governments as they interpret statutes, regulations, and the state and federal constitutions; (3) regulatory law, which is written by executive-branch bureaucracies, overseen by the courts and legislatures, and implements the intent of statutory law; and (4) administrative law, which is the set of legal rules and regulations to which the creation and enforcement of regulatory law must conform [3].

Medical practice in the United States is legally regulated mainly by the states, with federal regulation governing such matters as drug development and approval, dispensing controlled substances, and the oversight of research with human subjects. Thus, state law is the most relevant to informed consent. Most of the law on informed consent is common law, developed by various state courts. In some states, statutory law also regulates informed consent [3].

Ethics of informed consent

The ethics of informed consent concerns the justification of the physician's ethical obligations, as a matter of professional responsibility, to patients in communicating and making decisions with them. This justification has been developed on the basis of two ethical principles: beneficence and respect for autonomy (Box 1) [4].

In ethics generally, the ethical principle of beneficence requires one to act in a way that is expected reliably to produce the greater balance of benefits over harms in the lives of others [2]. To put this principle into clinical practice requires a reliable account of the benefits and harms relevant to the

---

Box 1. Two ethical principles in medical ethics

Beneficence obligates the physician to act in a way that is reliably expected to result in the greater balance of clinical goods over clinical harms for the patient, as judged from a rigorous, evidence-based clinical perspective.

Respect for autonomy obligates the physician to acknowledge the integrity of the patient's values and beliefs, to elicit her preferences, and to carry out that preferences, unless there are ethically compelling reasons for not doing so.

---

clinical care of the patient and of how those goods and harms should be reasonably balanced against each other when not all of them can be achieved in a particular clinical situation, such as a request for an elective Cesarean delivery [1]. In medical ethics, the ethical principle of beneficence requires the physician to act in a way that is reliably expected to produce the greater balance of clinical benefits over harms for the patient [1,2].

Expert, beneficence-based clinical judgment should conform to the requirements of evidence-based reasoning [5–8]. There is therefore a synergistic connection between evidence-based clinical reasoning and beneficence-based clinical reasoning. Technically possible clinical judgment for which there is an evidence base of expected net clinical benefit—the reduction of mortality and morbidity, the preservation of functional status, and the prevention and effective management of pain, distress, and suffering—is supported in beneficence-based clinical judgment. Technically possible clinical management that is supported in beneficence-based clinical judgment counts as medically reasonable clinical management. From the perspective of beneficence-based clinical judgment, not all technically possible clinical management is medically reasonable clinical management.

There is an inherent risk of paternalism in beneficence-based clinical judgment. Paternalism involves the interference with the patient's autonomy for beneficence-based reasons [1,2]. By this we mean that beneficence-based clinical judgment, if it is mistakenly considered to be the sole source of moral responsibility and therefore moral authority in medical care, invites the unwary physician to conclude that beneficence-based judgments can be imposed on the patient in violation of her autonomy. Paternalism is antithetical to the ethics of informed consent.

Paternalism should be distinguished from a paternalistic attitude (ie, an appropriately concerned attitude) toward patients. A paternalistic attitude of being concerned to protect patients from the potentially adverse consequences of their own decisions and behaviors is required by the professional virtue of compassion. A physician who did not care whether his or her patients were making bad decisions, clinically or personally, would exhibit an unprofessional indifference or disregard for the risks of such decisions and behaviors. Compassion thus motivates the physician in such cases to look after the patient [1]. This involves some risk of violating the patient's autonomy, but the alternative, a kind of moral abandonment, is worse from the perspective of professional ethics. When a patient's decision-making capacity seems to be impaired and she is making a clinically bad decision (ie, one that places her health seriously at risk), a paternalistic physician intervenes not to initiate treatment without consent but to recommend that the patient reconsider, to be alert to potential deficits in the decision-making capacity, and to initiate clinical evaluation of decision-making capacity, the components of which are discussed in greater detail below.

The informed consent process provides that the appropriate response to this inherent paternalism is for the physician to explain the diagnostic, therapeutic, and prognostic reasoning that leads to his or her expert clinical judgment about what is in the interest of the patient (ie, which technically possible forms of clinical management are medically reasonable) so that the patient can assess that judgment for herself or parents for themselves. This general rule can be put into clinical practice in the following way: The physician should disclose and explain to the patient the major factors of this reasoning process, including matters of uncertainty. In neither medical law nor medical ethics does this require that the patient be provided with a complete medical education [4]. In matters of clinical controversy (ie, in which there are competing medically reasonable ways to clinically manage the patient's problem), the physician should explain how and why other clinicians might reasonably differ from his or her clinical judgment. The physician should present a well reasoned response to this critique. In effect, the physician should take the patient through a lay version of evidence-based reasoning that is accessible to the layperson. The outcome of this process is that beneficence-based clinical judgments, by physicians and patients, take on a rigor that they sometimes lack, and the process of their formulation includes explaining them to the patient [1].

The principle of respect for autonomy

In contrast to the principle of beneficence, there is a strong emphasis in the literature of medical ethics on the ethical principle of respect for autonomy [1,2]. In medical ethics, this ethical principle requires one to acknowledge and carry out the value-based preferences of the adult, competent patient unless there is compelling ethical justification for not doing so. The pregnant patient increasingly brings to her medical care her own perspective on what is in her interest, as do parents on the care of their newborn child concerning what is in their child's interest. The ethical principle of respect for autonomy translates this fact into autonomy-based clinical judgment. Because each patient's perspective on her interests is a function of her values and beliefs, it is impossible to specify the benefits and harms of autonomy-based clinical judgment in advance. It would be inappropriate for the physician to do so because the definition of her benefits and harms and their balancing are the prerogative of the patient. Autonomy-based clinical judgment is strongly antipaternalistic [2].

To understand the moral demands of this principle, the ethical principle of respect for autonomy needs to be operationalized to make it relevant to and applicable in clinical practice. To accomplish this, seven steps of autonomous decision-making on the part of the patient have been identified (Box 2) [9].

The physician has a role in supporting the patient or parents as necessary by reason of impaired decision-making capacity or, as requested, to complete each of these components of autonomous decision making. The physician's role includes the obligations (1) to recognize the capacity of each patient to deal with medical information (and not to underestimate that capacity), to provide information (ie, disclose and explain all medically reasonable alternatives, such as those supported in beneficence-based clinical judgment), and to recognize the validity of the values and beliefs of the patient; (2) not to interfere with but, when necessary, to assist the patient in her evaluation and ranking of diagnostic and therapeutic alternatives for managing her condition; and (3) to elicit and implement the patient's value-based preference [1]. The ethics of informed consent, based on the

---

Box 2. Seven steps of autonomous decision making by patients and parents

1. The patient or parents attend to the information that the physician provides to her.
2. The patient or parents absorb, retain, and recall this information as needed in subsequent steps.
3. The patient or parents reason from present clinical events to their future, likely consequences (cognitive understanding).
4. The patient or parent believes that these consequences could happen to her, her fetus, her future child, or their infant (appreciation).
5. The patient or parents assess these consequences on the basis of their values and beliefs (evaluative understanding).
6. The patient or parents voluntary elect one of the medically reasonable alternatives offered or recommended or reject them all. "Voluntary" means that a decision is not subject to substantial control by external factors (other people) or internal factors (such as auditory hallucinations).
7. The patient or parents, when requested, explain their decision on the basis of their cognitive and evaluative understanding, with which the physician may disagree.

ethical principles of beneficence and respect for autonomy, results in an understanding of the informed consent process as comprising the elements listed in Box 3.

Box 3. The physician's and the patient's or parents' roles in the informed consent process

The physician's initial role
1. The physician, following the intellectual discipline of evidence-based reasoning, forms an expert, beneficence-based clinical judgment about which technically possible alternatives for clinically managing the patient's problem are medically reasonable.
2. The physician offers these medically reasonable alternatives to the patient or parents, explains the nature of each, and provides information about each medically reasonable alternative's expected clinical benefits and clinical risks (guided by rigorous clinical judgment about what is salient for future treatment planning for the patient).
3. The physician recommends an alternative when it is the only medically reasonable alternative or when evidence-based reasoning supports it as the better or best among two or more medically reasonable alternatives.
4. The physician encourages the patient or parents to ask questions and addresses the patient's or parents' questions respectfully and thoroughly.

The patient's or parents' role
5. The patient or parents complete the steps of autonomous decision making (see Box 2).

The physician's continuing role
6. The physician should elicit the patient's or parents' decision about acceptance of a medically reasonable alternative.
7. The physician implements that decision. When organizational policy requires a signed consent form or operative or intervention permit, the patient's or parents' formal approval and signature should be obtained.

The physician's concluding role
8. The progress notes in the patient's record should summarize steps 1 through 6. Signed consent forms should be part of the patient's record.

Law of informed consent

In the United States, the legal obligations of the physician regarding informed consent were established in a series of court cases during the twentieth century that first established the concept of simple consent and then the concept of informed consent [4]. Most of the legal literature on informed consent assumes that the law shaped medical practice, not ethics. Recent historical scholarship has called this assumption into question. The more plausible account is that physicians developed consent practices as early as the seventeenth century, during which British surgeons drew contracts with patients for surgical management of their problems [10]. This was followed in the eighteenth century by the argument of the Scottish physician-ethicist John Gregory (1724–1773) of Edinburgh that the patient has a right to speak in matters that concern his or her own life and health and that the physician should take seriously the expressed preferences of patients [11]. In nineteenth-century Brooklyn, the gynecologist Alexander Skene (d. 1900) developed what twentieth-century law and medical ethics would recognize and endorse as informed consent practices for gynecologic surgery [12]. The emerging interpretation of this history is that the common law of informed consent was influenced by emerging best ethical practices of informed consent. This interpretation challenges the interpretation common in the literature on informed consent that the law invented the concept of informed consent and required medical practice to conform to it.

Simple consent

In 1914, Schloendorff v The Society of The New York Hospital established the concept of simple consent (ie, whether the patient says "yes" or "no" to medical intervention) [13]. In the medical and bioethics literature, this decision is quoted: "Every human being of adult years and sound mind has the right to determine what shall be done with his body, and a surgeon who performs an operation without his patient's consent commits an assault for which he is liable in damages" [13]. The legal requirement of consent evolved to include disclosure of information sufficient to enable patients to make informed decisions about whether to say "yes" or "no" to medical intervention (ie, simple consent) [4].

Informed consent

The physician's obligation to provide information adequate for the patient to make an informed decision added to the concept of simple consent, which was still required, the concept of informed consent. Informed consent requires the physician first to disclose information to the patient and then to obtain the patient'ss acceptance or refusal. Standards that should guide the physician in fulfilling his or her disclosure obligation to the patient become central concerns [4]. Two legal standards have emerged to guide such disclosure. The professional community standard, adopted in the minority of the states, defines adequate disclosure in the context of what the relevantly trained and experienced physician tells patients [4]. The reasonable person standard, which has been adopted by most states, goes further and requires the physician to disclose "material" information, what any patient in the patient's condition needs to know, and what the lay person of average sophistication should not be expected to know [4]. A rule of thumb for translating the reasonable person standard into clinical practice is for the physician to identify clinically salient information about the patient's condition and its management and then provide this information to the patient [14]. This reasonable person standard has emerged as the ethical standard [1,2], and perinatologists should adopt it. On this standard, the physician should disclose to the patient her or the pregnant woman's, the fetus', or the infant's diagnosis (including differential diagnosis when that is all that is known), the medically reasonable alternatives to diagnose and manage the patient's condition, and the short-term and long-term benefits and risks of each alternative.

The main justification for the reasonable person standard becoming the preferred ethical standard is the history of systematic underdisclosure of information to patients when physicians successfully established that they met the professional community standard of disclosure [4]. Prominent examples that led state and federal courts to reject the professional community standard in favor of the reasonable person standard included nondisclosure of the risks of cobalt radiation therapy [15] and nondisclosure of the risk of paralyzing injury from falls in the immediate postoperative period after a laminectomy [16]. The emergence of the reasonable person standard as the dominant legal and accepted ethical standard is a function of the stark recognition of the shortcomings of the professional community standard and its tendency toward paternalism, resulting in failure to disclose clinically salient information to patients [4].

A major difference between the law and ethics of informed consent

There is a major difference between the law and ethics of informed consent when it comes to the patient's role in the decision-making process. The law of informed consent developed in tort actions brought by patients against physicians. Because the allegations were that the physician had failed in a professional obligation to the patient, little attention was paid by the courts to the patient's role in decision making with her physician. In one prominent and influential federal court ruling, the court stated that, in response to disclosure by the physician satisfying the reasonable person standard, "rough understanding" by the patient will do [16].

This may be an ethically satisfactory standard for the patient's role when it comes to understanding clear and stark risks, such as paralyzing injury from falls after a laminectomy procedure. As clinical matters become more complex, the cognitive demands on the patient increase. This is especially the case in perinatal medicine, in which pregnant women are presented with complex, sometimes uncertain information about their own or a fetus' diagnosis and must make judgments about how to balance their own interests and those of the fetus(es). Parents of newborn infants who have major medical problems confront similarly complex and cognitively demanding decisions. As the cognitive demands of decision making by the patient increase, the importance of the physician's role in assisting the patient to exercise her capacity for autonomous decision making increases. Increasing cognitive demands should not be regarded by the physician as a justification for diminishing the patient's or parent's role in decision making.

Responding to a patient's refusal

Sometimes a patient refuses to authorize any of the medically reasonable alternatives for the clinical management of her problem or condition. The first response of the physician should be not to take such refusal personally or to think badly of the patient or parents. The physician should assume that, based on the information that the woman or parents have and their evaluation of it, they have a good reason for their refusal. The information that she or they have, however, may be incomplete or inaccurate. To address this problem, the physician should take the patient or parents through the decision-making process again but should start the process with a request that the patient or parents explain their current understanding of the patient's or child's condition, the medically reasonable alternatives for managing it clinically, and the benefits and risks of each alternative. The physician should be attentive to incomplete or inaccurate cognitive understanding and, in a respectful and supportive fashion, should correct these deficits and assist the patient or parents to integrate this corrected or new information into their cognitive understanding. The patient or parents should be asked to consider this corrected information and their decision.

If the patient or parents persist in their refusal, the physician should ask them what their goals are for themselves, or in the case of a pregnant women for her child. One way to do so is to ask, "As you consider this new information, what is important for you in your own/your child's care?" The physician should consider the values expressed in response to this question and ask himself or herself whether any of those values—it need be all of them—support any of the medically reasonable alternatives. When that is the case, the physician should not hesitate to point this out respectfully and ask the patient or parents what she or they think about this judgment. In the medical ethics literature, this is known as respectful persuasion—asking the patient or parents to reconsider their refusal based on their own expressed values. This is different from paternalism in response to refusal, in which the physician attempts to impose on the pregnant woman or parents a view of what their values ought to be [1].

When attempts to have the patient or parents reconsider refusal (ie, when respectful persuasion fails to alter the refusal and the patient or parents continue refuse to accept any of the alternatives supported in beneficence-based clinical judgment), the physician is ethically and legally obligated to engage in what is known as "informed refusal." This legal and ethical obligation arises from the 1980 case of Truman v Thomas from California [17]. Dr. Thomas had delivered several of Mrs. Truman's babies and, on the delivery of her last child, had recommended that she have a Pap smear. She refused to have this test until she could pay for it and did not accept Dr. Thomas's offer to perform it without charge. Mrs. Truman later presented to Dr. Thomas with advanced cervical cancer, from which she died. In the malpractice action brought by her survivors, Dr. Thomas stated that, although they were of clinical concern to him in the management of Mrs. Truman, he did not tell Mrs. Truman of the risks of having detectable presymptomatic changes in her cervix indicative of cervical cancer or that he was concerned that she could die from such disease. The California Supreme Court ruled that, because risks were of clinical salience to Dr. Thomas—they were the motivation for his offering the Pap smear—he should have informed Mrs. Thomas about these risks so that her refusal would be informed. This case changed practice and introduced the concept of informed refusal into medical law and ethics.

The ethical and legal obligation of the physician in the matter of informed refusal is clear and, as a matter of strict legal obligation, should always be fulfilled. It is not difficult to fulfill. The patient should be informed about the medical risks that she is taking in her refusal of medically reasonable alternatives for the management of her condition, and parents should be told the same about their refusal of an infant's appropriate clinical management. The risks to be disclosed are those that are salient in clinical judgment: If they are important to the physician (ie, motivating the offering or recommending of the diagnostic test or therapy), they are salient. This discussion, detailing the disclosure of the risks of refusal, should be thoroughly documented in the patient's chart.

This is all that the law requires. Good ethical practice requires that this disclosure be followed by a recommendation that the patient reconsider her refusal. Perhaps the disclosure of the risks the patient is taking will help to persuade her to reconsider her refusal. This approach avoids the need to abandon the patient, keeps lines of communication open, and sends a powerful signal of concern by the physician to the patient about the medical gravity of her refusal.

Summary

The physician's obligations and role and the patient's or parent's decision making about medical care play a central role in forming a strong physician–patient or physician–parent relationship. Although the law of informed consent is important, especially concerning informed refusal, ethics is more important. This is because the law of informed consent focuses almost exclusively on the physician's disclosure obligations to the patient. Ethics goes further and describes meaningful roles for the physician and patient and for the physician and parents in the decision-making process about medical care. Meeting the ethical standards of informed consent satisfies legal obligations and helps to build a strong therapeutic alliance with the pregnant woman and parents, which is essential for supporting them through the demanding clinical decisions that arise in perinatal medicine. We hope that the reader now appreciates the legal and ethical dimensions are essential to excellent patient. Informed consent should no longer be treated in clinical practice in a perfunctory, bureaucratic fashion.

References

[1] McCullough LB, Chervenak FA. Ethics in obstetrics and gynecology. New York: Oxford University Press; 1994.

[2] Beauchamp TL, Childress JF. Principles of biomedical ethics. 5th edition. New York: Oxford University Press; 2001.

[3] Sanbar SS, American College of Legal Medicine Textbook Committee. Legal medicine. Mosby: Philadelphia; 2004.

[4] Faden RR, Beauchamp TL. A history and theory of informed consent. New York: Oxford University Press; 1986.

[5] Guyatt GH, Sackett DL, Cook DJ. Users' guide to the medical literature: II. How to use an article about therapy or prevention. A. Are the results of the study valid? JAMA 1993;270: 2598–601.

[6] Guyatt GH, Sackett DL, Cook DJ. Users' guide to the medical literature: II. How to use an article about therapy or prevention. B. What were the results and will they help me in caring for my patients? JAMA 1994;271:59–63.

[7] Wilson MC, Hayward RS, Tunis SR, et al. Users' guides to the medical literature: VIII. How to use clinical practice guidelines. A. Are the recommendations valid? JAMA 1995;274:570–4.

[8] Wilson MC, Hayward RS, Tunis SR, et al. Users' guides to the medical literature: VIII. How to use clinical practice guidelines. B. What are the recommendations and will they help you in caring for your patients? JAMA 1995;274:1630–2.

[9] McCullough LB, Coverdale JH, Chervenak FA. Ethical challenges of decision making with pregnant patients who have schizophrenia. Am J Obstet Gynecol 2002;187:696–702.

[10] Wear A. Medical ethics in early modern England. In: Wear A, Geyer-Kordesch J, French P, editors. Doctors and ethics: the earlier historical setting of professional ethics. Amsterdam (The Netherlands): Rodopi; 1993. p. 98–130.

[11] McCullough LB. John Gregory's invention of professional medical ethics and the profession of medicine. Dordrecht (The Netherlands): Kluwer Academic Publishers; 1998.

[12] Powderly K. Patient consent and negotiation in the gynecological practice of Alexander J.C. Skene 1863–1900. J Med Philos 2000;25:12–27.

[13] Schloendorff v The Society of The New York Hospital, 211 N.Y. 125, 126, 105 N.E. 92, 93 (1914).

[14] Wear S. Informed consent: patient autonomy and clinician beneficence within health care. 2nd edition. Washington, DC: Georgetown University Press; 1998.

[15] Natanson v Kline, 186 Kan. 393, 350 P.2d 1093, 354 P.2d 670 (1960).

[16] Canterbury v Spence, 464 F.2d 772, 775 (D.C Cir. 1972).

[17] Truman v Thomas 611 P.2d 902 (Cal. 1980).

ELSEVIER
SAUNDERS

CLINICS IN
PERINATOLOGY

Clin Perinatol 34 (2007) 287–297

Medical Legal Issues in Prenatal Diagnosis

Roger D. Klein, MD, JD,
Maurice J. Mahoney, MD, JD*

*Department of Genetics, Yale University School of Medicine, P.O. Box 208005,
New Haven, CT 06520-8005, USA*

Prenatal diagnostic testing offers parents the option of avoiding the physical suffering and emotional trauma that attends the birth of children who have severe, debilitating diseases, such as Tay-Sachs, Canavan, ornithine transcarbamylase deficiency, and Down syndrome. In addition, prenatal diagnosis can alert families and health care providers of the need to prepare for the delivery of a compromised child. Finally, in utero diagnostics increasingly help guide physicians and parents or present physicians and parents with opportunities for fetal therapy [1–5]. Although prenatal diagnostic testing encompasses a broad range of clinical diagnostic investigations for genetic and nongenetic conditions, the focus of this article is on the legal issues surrounding DNA-based prenatal testing for inherited conditions. Many principles discussed in this article are applicable to prenatal diagnosis performed for other reasons.

After the demonstration by Steele and Breg [6] in 1966 that chromosomes could be analyzed from cultured amniotic fluid cells, technical advances in cytogenetics, ultrasonography, clinical chemistry, biochemical genetics, and molecular diagnostics, together with legal changes stemming from the Supreme Court's decision in Roe v Wade [7], brought about dramatic growth in the implementation of prenatal diagnosis and screening in clinical obstetrics practice. Screening tests, most often using a pregnant woman's blood, enable more precise statements about risks of certain fetal diseases or defects. Ultrasonography or other imaging techniques may establish a fetal diagnosis or may reveal abnormal anatomy that generates an extensive differential diagnosis. Invasive procedures, like amniocentesis and chorionic villus sampling (CVS), offer definitive diagnoses and have low complication rates.

* Corresponding author.
E-mail address: maurice.mahoney@yale.edu (M.J. Mahoney).

0095-5108/07/$ - see front matter © 2007 Elsevier Inc. All rights reserved.
doi:10.1016/j.clp.2007.03.006   *perinatology.theclinics.com*

Although testing for Down syndrome and other aneuploidies in women of advanced maternal age remains the most common indication for invasive prenatal testing, in utero diagnosis of a growing list of diseases and anomalies by analysis of fetal DNA is increasing in frequency [8]. The current introduction of array comparative genomic hybridization techniques is quickly expanding the diagnosis of small chromosomal abnormalities [9]. Future recommendations to offer widespread DNA-based carrier assessment and prenatal testing similar to those that have been published for cystic fibrosis [10] and fragile X syndrome [11] will likely accelerate the trend toward greater reliance on the use of molecular diagnostic techniques for prenatal diagnosis. Developments in technology have made clinical mutation detection from blood and other human tissues routine [12]. In the near future, noninvasive ways to accomplish DNA-based fetal genetic testing [13,14] will greatly enhance the importance of prenatal diagnostics to obstetricians, geneticists, primary care physicians, pathologists, and other clinical laboratory physicians.

The legal and ethical issues associated with prenatal diagnosis are complex and evolving. It will increasingly be necessary for practitioners to become informed about, and stay abreast of changes in, laws affecting the use of prenatal diagnosis. Key legal areas of concern in the United States include the requirements for informed consent and prenatal genetic counseling, definitions of negligent practice (particularly in relation to wrongful birth and wrongful life lawsuits), and genetic discrimination.

Informed consent

The modern concept of informed consent evolved from the law of "battery" [15]. Battery is defined as an intentional, nonconsensual, offensive touching of another person [16]. In part because of its historical roots, most physicians are familiar with the need to obtain informed consent before performing invasive diagnostic or therapeutic procedures. The requirement for informed consent extends to the provision of all medical care, including diagnostic laboratory testing. Battery has largely been supplanted by negligence (ie, medical malpractice) as a basis for litigation over the alleged failure of a physician to obtain informed consent. This is likely because most such claims are raised in conjunction with other allegations of substandard care, none of which reflects the deliberate intent to injure patient plaintiffs.

It is conceivable that a patient who was injured during CVS, for example, could rely on a battery theory if she alleges that the procedure was unnecessarily performed. A battery claim could also be raised by a patient who argues that the scope of diagnostic testing performed on her behalf exceeded that for which she gave consent. For example, if a patient who has a family history of Huntington disease underwent CVS for reasons unrelated to that disorder, and testing for Huntington Disease was mistakenly performed on the fetal tissue without the patient's consent, she could potentially argue battery as one of her claims in a lawsuit against the ordering provider.

Some commentators have argued that the immutable, highly personal, and powerfully predictive nature of the information obtained from DNA-based diagnostic tests mandates that performance of these tests and protection of test results receive regulatory and legal considerations above and beyond those already accorded clinical laboratory testing and health care information generally [17,18]. Similar concerns have prompted several states to enact statutes that specifically require informed consent before genetic testing is undertaken [19].

New York Civil Rights Law 79-1(2)(a), for example, in part reads: "No person shall perform a genetic test on a biological sample taken from an individual without the prior written informed consent of such individual..." [20]. The New York statute and those of some other states specify minimum content for requisite written consent forms. Section 34-14-22 of the South Dakota Codified Laws [21] mandates use of a written form that includes:

The nature and purpose of the predictive genetic test

The effectiveness and limitations of the predictive genetic test

The implications of taking the predictive genetic test, including the medical risks and benefits

The future uses of the sample taken from the person tested to conduct the predictive genetic test and the information obtained from the predictive genetic test

The meaning of the predictive genetic test results and the procedure for providing notice of the results to the person tested

A listing of who will have access to the sample taken from the person tested to conduct the predictive genetic test and the information obtained from the predictive genetic test and the person's right to confidential treatment of the sample and the information

Consent for genetic testing, like other medical care, must truly be "informed." In fact, physicians are more commonly accused of providing insufficient information than no information at all. Obstetricians have a duty to offer general, and in many cases patient-specific, prenatal diagnostic testing and prenatal genetic counseling. Therefore, obstetricians who neglect to document that they have conveyed and that the patient has understood essential information about a test they have ordered leave themselves open to allegations that they failed to obtain informed consent for the testing. This information may include the risks of having an infant who has the disease in question, its probable course, the risks and limitations of test procedures used, the length of time required to complete testing, the costs of testing, the patient's reproductive options, and potential therapies for the condition for which investigation is pursued.

An obstetrical provider is obligated to obtain thorough patient, family, and ethnic histories and to engage in discussions or evaluations for disorders for which prospective parents are at heightened risk. If the provider fails to do so and an infant manifests such a disorder, he or she risks allegations that care was rendered without informed consent [22]. It is not essential that obstetricians provide all or even the majority of the required genetic counseling; obstetricians can refer patients to genetics professionals, such as medical geneticists or genetic counselors.

Genetic counseling

Prenatal genetic counseling is intended to provide patients with sufficient information to enable them to make informed, autonomous decisions regarding their reproductive decisions. As such, some argue that it should be nondirective [23]. Complete nondirectiveness is difficult to achieve in practice, and challenges to this concept emanate from several sources.

First, patients often have a limited understanding of and experience with the complex, highly technical topics presented to them. Second, information with significant emotional connotations must be conveyed to patients within limited time frames and in circumstances under which patients may feel psychologically overwhelmed. Third, as with other forms of medical practice, there is a tendency for many patients to desire, request, or attempt to extract guidance from an experienced, trusted professional in an area in which they feel uncomfortable and poorly equipped to make decisions. Subtle changes in tone of voice, body language, and manner of presentation, as with other human communication, can signal personal feelings of the practitioner with respect to the topic at hand. Finally, the superior medical knowledge of the practitioner relative to the patient, the often complex nature of genetics problems, and the limited time patients and providers have together necessitate that the provider filter the information he or she delivers to the patient. The information given to individual patients requires judgment upon which personal beliefs of the practitioner can easily encroach. Nevertheless, practitioners do have a professional, ethical, and perhaps at times an enforceable legal duty to strive toward nondirectiveness during patient genetic counseling.

Wrongful birth and wrongful life (negligence)

Negligence, referred to in the medical context as "medical malpractice," refers to substandard performance by a medical practitioner. A lawsuit for medical malpractice requires that the defendant physician have a duty to render appropriate medical care to the plaintiff. The lawsuit must allege that breach of this duty by the defendant's substandard medical practice caused a legally compensable injury to the plaintiff.

Potential medical malpractice liability can arise from recognized complications of amniocentesis or CVS, such as maternal infection, fetal loss or injury, or the development of anti-D antibodies in an Rh-negative mother who was not administered postprocedure Rh immune globulin. To give rise to legal liability, such complications must result from negligence by the provider. Otherwise, according to the law, patients bear the risk of bad outcomes associated with medical care.

The duty to provide prenatal testing and counseling has also spawned less straightforward variants on the medical malpractice theme. Lawsuits for "wrongful birth" and "wrongful life" arise out of the birth of an impaired child who, it is claimed, would have been aborted or not conceived but for the negligence of the provider. As the Alabama Supreme Court stated in the case of Keel v Banach [24]:

> The nature of the tort of wrongful birth has nothing to do with whether a defendant caused the injury or harm to the child, but rather, with whether the defendant's negligence was the proximate cause of the parents' being deprived of the option of avoiding a conception or, in the case of pregnancy, making an informed and meaningful decision either to terminate the pregnancy or to give birth to a potentially defective child.

The usual basis for a wrongful birth or wrongful life lawsuit is the physician's failure to properly diagnose a fetal abnormality or disease predisposition or to inform prospective parents of the risks thereof under circumstances in which this omission results in the birth of a diseased or disabled child.

Wrongful birth and wrongful life lawsuits stem from the identical set of facts and circumstances. They differ in that the parents are the plaintiffs in wrongful birth lawsuits, whereas wrongful life suits are filed on behalf of the disabled child. In wrongful birth lawsuits, parents argue that if they had been adequately informed of their reproductive risks, they would have taken steps to prevent the pregnancy or birth of the impaired child. In wrongful life suits, the child or a legal representative claims that he or she would be better off having not been born than living with the present disability. The child avers that but for the negligence of the treating physician, he or she would not have had to endure the suffering that has accompanied the condition. In neither type of lawsuit do plaintiffs accuse their physicians of causing the child's disability. Instead, they argue that they are entitled to compensation because, absent the provider's negligence, the child would not have been born.

Wrongful birth and wrongful life claims were universally rejected by courts until the late 1960s under the reasoning that it was against public policy to recognize the birth of any infant as injury. For example, in the often cited case of Gleitman v Cosgrove [25], Sandra Gleitman alleged that her physician, Dr. Robert Cosgrove, Jr., failed to inform her that her first-trimester rubella infection could produce birth defects in her child. After their son was found to be blind and deaf, Mrs. Gleitman and her husband filed malpractice suits against Dr. Cosgrove and another physician on their own behalf and on behalf of their affected child. The Gleitmans argued that the negligent failure of her physicians to inform Mrs. Gleitman of the potential consequences of her rubella infection deprived her of the possibility of terminating her pregnancy.

The New Jersey Supreme Court refused to allow the wrongful life or wrongful birth claims to proceed, stating:

> We are not faced here with the necessity of balancing the mother's life against that of her child. The sanctity of the single human life is the decisive factor in this suit in tort. Eugenic considerations are not controlling. We are not talking here about the breeding of prize cattle. It may have been easier for the mother and less expensive for the father to have terminated the life of their child while he was an embryo, but these alleged detriments cannot stand against the preciousness of the single human life to support a remedy in tort.

This 1967 case was decided before the United States Supreme Court's landmark 1973 decision in Roe v Wade [7], which created a constitutional right to undergo an abortion. Twelve years later, the New Jersey Supreme Court explicitly relied in part on Roe when it reversed its holding in Gleitman with respect to wrongful birth suits. In Berman v Allen [26], a 38-year-old mother claimed to have given birth to a son with Down syndrome because she was not offered amniocentesis, the results of which would have caused her to abort the child. The Court in its opinion wrote:

> The Supreme Court's ruling in Roe v. Wade, supra, clearly established that a woman possesses a constitutional right to decide whether her fetus should be aborted, at least during the first trimester of pregnancy. Public policy now supports, rather than militates against, the proposition that she not be impermissibly denied a meaningful opportunity to make that decision.

Thus, changes in the law and in social and culture mores have combined with technologic and medical advances in prenatal diagnostics to encourage increased receptivity of courts to wrongful birth, if not wrongful life, lawsuits. This has led to a dramatic expansion in the number of such lawsuits filed.

Wrongful life lawsuits continue to meet with limited success. This is at least in part because these suits make it difficult for courts to avoid confronting a value judgment of whether or not never having been born is preferable to life with the handicap, impairment, or disease at issue. As the New York Court of Appeals stated in the well known case of Becker v Schwartz [27]:

> Whether it is better never to have been born at all than to have been born with even gross deficiencies is a mystery more properly left to the philosophers and the theologians. Surely the law can assert no competence to resolve the issue, particularly in view of the very nearly uniform high value

which the law and mankind have placed on human life, rather than its absence…Simply put, a cause of action brought on behalf of an infant seeking recovery for wrongful life demands a calculation of damages dependent upon a comparison between the Hobson's choice of life in an impaired state and nonexistence. This comparison the law is not equipped to make.

There is concern that allowing wrongful life claims against physicians will prompt analogous claims against parents who, despite having been informed of the likelihood of giving birth to a severely impaired child, knowingly waived their opportunity to abort the fetus. This point was acknowledged by a California state appeals court in Curlender v Bio-Science Laboratories [28], one of the few cases that has held wrongful life to be a valid claim. In Curlender, a lawsuit filed on behalf of an infant who had Tay-Sachs disease against a diagnostic laboratory that performed faulty carrier testing on his parents, the court wrote:

> One of the fears expressed in the decisional law is that, once it is determined that such infants have rights cognizable at law, nothing would prevent such a plaintiff from bringing suit against its own parents for allowing the plaintiff to be born…If a case arose where, despite due care by the medical profession in transmitting the necessary warnings, parents made a conscious choice to proceed with a pregnancy, with full knowledge that a seriously impaired infant would be born…we see no sound public policy which should protect those parents from being answerable for the pain, suffering and misery which they have wrought upon their offspring.

Despite their controversy, wrongful life lawsuits have been allowed to proceed by the highest courts in California [29], New Jersey [30], and Washington [31].

In contrast to wrongful life claims, wrongful birth lawsuits have met with a much higher degree of success, with a majority of jurisdictions allowing these claims. New York's highest court in Becker v Schwartz denied the plaintiff's claim for wrongful life. In this seminal case, the court also held that an obstetrician could be found liable for failing to advise 37-year-old Doris Becker of her increased risk of delivering a child with Down syndrome and for neglecting to offer her amniocentesis to diagnose the condition in her son. The Court allowed Becker to sue for the expenses relating to the care and treatment of the child. The court refused to permit the Beckers to recover damages for emotional or psychic injury suffered in response to the birth of their handicapped son.

A minority of courts have taken a contrary view of wrongful birth suits. In Azzolino v Dingfelder [32], the North Carolina Supreme Court declined to allow a wrongful birth suit to go forward. In this case, the parents of a child born with Down syndrome alleged that their caregivers, a nurse practitioner and her supervising obstetrician, were negligent in failing to offer them genetic counseling and amniocentesis. Were it not for their providers' malpractice, the plaintiffs claimed, they would not have given birth to their child, whom they would have aborted. The court, in refusing to accept this argument, wrote:

> [S]uch a step requires a view of human life previously unknown to the law of this jurisdiction. We are unwilling to take any such step because we are unwilling to say that life, even life with severe defects, may ever amount to a legal injury.

A few states have passed statutes that prohibit wrongful birth and wrongful life lawsuits against health care providers. Although such statutes have been challenged on constitutional grounds as encumbrances on procreative rights, this argument has yet to be accepted by any court.

Although the majority view has been consistent in upholding the legality of wrongful birth lawsuits, courts have handled the issue of damages in varying and inconsistent ways. Damages have been awarded based on varying combinations of the expenses that are directly attributable to the physician's negligence. These include the costs of the continued pregnancy, the delivery, and those extraordinary medical costs incurred solely as a result of the child's disability. In some jurisdictions, damages have been awarded to the parents for emotional pain and suffering. A court may also permit a damage award for emotional injuries but must offset them with an estimate of the disabled child's positive value to the family. The law in this area can be murky and varies based on the state in which a provider practices.

Providers have professional and legal responsibilities to adequately inform patients of potential risks of having children who have genetic or congenital anomalies, to offer genetic or other testing when available and appropriate, and to properly convey the results of diagnostic evaluations. Given the rapid advances that are occurring in prenatal diagnostic techniques and the current trend toward allowing plaintiffs compensation in wrongful birth lawsuits, key questions for providers are: How much information are we legally obligated to present to patients? What do we need to tell them about reproductive risks and potential diagnostic and therapeutic options? What diseases must we discuss? What services must we offer them? Molecular test offerings now include symptom, disease, and ethnically determined panels. Must all pregnant Ashkenazi Jews and their partners be offered the complete "Ashkenazi Jewish" test panel?

In this era of rapid development of molecular genetic tests, there are no definitive answers to these questions. We are obligated to counsel and offer screening for relatively common genetic maladies, such as cystic fibrosis, and for a standard body of infectious diseases. Further, we are obliged to warn parents about and offer evaluation for well known ethnically, racially, and age-related risks. Finally, patient-specific risks, based on personal, family, and pregnancy histories, must be discussed. Clinicians may also be held at least partially responsible for errors in specimen handling and sample mix-ups that occur before delivery to the diagnostic laboratory. They also have legal responsibilities to properly use diagnostic tests and accurately interpret and convey their results. They can share responsibility for performance of the laboratory itself if they know or should recognize or suspect that there has been an error in the reported laboratory results.

Under traditional negligence principles, a physician's obligations are to adhere to the prevailing standard of medical practice. According to this view, what one must do is primarily determined by what one's peers do. In malpractice suits, courts need not rely exclusively on professionally determined standards. For example, a court could choose to impose a "patient-centric" perspective on the physician's obligation to provide information to the patient. By this analysis, liability could turn on whether or not the information would likely be important to a reasonable person in the patient's position. If the answer is yes, the physician was responsible for disclosing it. As our ability to perform predictive genetic testing for multifactorial disease, behavioral traits, or aptitudes and abilities improves, it remains to be seen where the lines of responsibility will be drawn. Will the costs of testing and therapy or the availability of insurance coverage influence the standards to which we are held?

It seems possible that our legal duty will expand from a predominantly medically determined standard of care to one that incorporates greater non-medical input. Society as a whole may help us decide how to deal with milder diseases or those that express in adulthood in the prenatal setting. This contribution would address the profound moral and ethical questions raised by prenatal genetic testing and reflect contemporary mores, beliefs, and aspirations. Perhaps a general consensus will help draw the line at which parents may no longer claim a child is so damaged that they would have aborted him or her.

Genetic discrimination

Because prenatal genetic testing reveals information about the fetus and the parents, some parents may be reluctant to undergo prenatal genetic testing out of fear of discrimination by employers or insurers. These are legitimate concerns, although they have not proved to be significant problems for most people. The majority of states have enacted laws that outlaw the use of genetic tests in determining eligibility for health insurance or its costs. These prohibitions do not apply to life or disability insurance. Thirty-four states have enacted laws banning discrimination in employment based on the results of genetic testing. In addition, the Equal Employment Opportunity Commission interprets the Americans with Disabilities Act to include the inherited predisposition to disease. Finally, under HIPAA, group health insurers are prohibited from applying "pre-existing condition" exclusions to genetic conditions diagnosed solely on the basis of genetic testing, as opposed to symptoms.

We recommend that practitioners familiarize themselves with the relevant statutes within their respective states and discuss their implications with hospital or other counsel to effectively address patient concerns about these issues. The Genetic Information Nondiscrimination Act, which limits the use of "genetic information" by health insurance companies and employers, has previously passed in the US Senate. A companion bill, H.R. 493, passed in the US House of Representatives in April 2007 at the time of this writing. The President was expect to sign the bill into law after the two versions were reconciled. H.R. 493 defines genetic information as information about an individual's genetic tests and those of his or her family members as "the occurrence of a disease or disorder in family members of the individual."

Summary

Advances in technology and genetic knowledge are likely to enhance the importance of prenatal testing in future obstetrics practice. Because of the complexity of the ethical, legal, and social issues associated with prenatal diagnostic testing, it will increasingly be necessary for providers to understand the laws that affect the use of prenatal diagnostic testing. The most important of these include the provider's duty to obtain informed consent from and offer prenatal genetic counseling to patients, the standards for establishing negligence, and genetic discrimination.

References

[1] Nimkarn S, New MI. Prenatal diagnosis and treatment of congenital adrenal hyperplasia. Horm Res 2006;67:53–60.
[2] Wilson RD, Hedrick HL, Liechty KW, et al. Cystic adenomatoid malformation of the lung: review of genetics, prenatal diagnosis, and in utero treatment. Am J Med Genet A 2006;140: 151–5.
[3] Cuneo BF, Ovadia M, Strasburger JF, et al. Prenatal diagnosis and in utero treatment of torsades de pointes associated with congenital long QT syndrome. Am J Cardiol 2003;91: 1395–8.
[4] Rahbar R, Vogel A, Myers LB, et al. Fetal surgery in otolaryngology: a new era in the diagnosis and management of fetal airway obstruction because of advances in prenatal imaging. Arch Otolaryngol Head Neck Surg 2005;131:393–8.
[5] Coutelle C, Themis M, Waddington SN, et al. Gene therapy progress and prospects: fetal gene therapy–first proofs of concept–some adverse effects. Gene Ther 2005;1601–7.
[6] Steele MW, Breg WR. Chromosome analysis of human amniotic-fluid cells. Lancet 1966;1: 383–5.
[7] Roe v Wade, 410 U.S. 113 (1973).
[8] Wilson RD. Amniocentesis and chorionic villus sampling. Curr Opin Obstet Gynecol 2000; 12:81–6.
[9] Sahoo T, Cheung SW, Ward P, et al. Prenatal diagnosis of chromosomal abnormalities using array-based comparative genomic hybridization. Genet Med 2006;8:719–27.
[10] ACOG committee opinion. No. 325: update on carrier screening for cystic fibrosis. Obstet Gynecol 2005;106:1465–8.

[11] ACOG committee opinion. No. 338: screening for fragile X syndrome. Obstet Gynecol 2006; 107:1483–5.

[12] Klein RD, Kant JA. Opportunity knocks: the pathologist as laboratory genetics consultant. Arch Pathol Lab Med 2006;130:1603–4.

[13] Bianchi DW, Hanson J. Sharpening the tools: a summary of a National Institutes of Health workshop on new technologies for detection of fetal cells in maternal blood for early prenatal diagnosis. J Matern Fetal Med 2006;19:199–207.

[14] Bianchi DW, Wataganara T, Lapaire O, et al. Fetal nucleic acids in maternal body fluids. Ann NY Acad Sci 2006;1075:63–73.

[15] Noah L. Informed consent and the elusive dichotomy between standard and experimental therapy. Am J Law Med 2002;28:361–408.

[16] Intentional Interference with the Person § 9. Battery. In: Keeton WP, Dobbs DB, Keeton RE, et al, editors. Prosser and Keeton on torts. 5th edition. St. Paul (MN): West Publishing Co.; 1984. p. 39–43.

[17] Hudson KL. Genetic testing oversight. Science 2006;313:1853.

[18] Slaughter LM. Genetic testing and discrimination: how private is your information? Stanford Law Pol Rev 2006;17:67–81.

[19] Ariz. Rev. Stat. § 12–2803 (2005); Mich. Comp. Laws Serv. § 333.17020 (LexisNexis 2005); Neb. Rev. Stat. Ann.§ 71-71,104.01 (LexisNexis 2006); N.Y. Civ. R. Law § 79-l, (Consol. 2006); Or. Rev. Stat. 678(2005); S.C. Code Ann.§ 38-93-40 (2005); S.D. Codified Laws § 34-14-22 (2006).

[20] N.Y. Civ. R. Law § 79-l, (Consol. 2006).

[21] S.D., Codified Laws § 34-14-22 (2006).

[22] See e.g., Lininger v Eisenbaum, 764 P.2d 1202, 1214 (Colo. 1988) (Mullarkey J., dissenting); Smith v. Cote, 513 A.2d 341 (N.H. 1986).

[23] Harper PS. Practical genetic counselling. 6th edition. London: Arnold; 2004. p. 3–20.

[24] Keel v Banach, 624 So.2d 1022, 1029 (Ala. 1993).

[25] Gleitman v Cosgrove, 227 A.2d 689 (N.J. 1967).

[26] Berman v Allen, 404 A.2d 8 (N.J. 1979).

[27] Becker v Schwartz, 386 N.E.2d 807 (N.Y. 1978).

[28] Curlender v Bio-Science Laboratories, 106 Cal.App.3d 811 (1980).

[29] Turpin v Sortini, 643 P.2d 954 (Cal. 1982).

[30] Procanik v Cillo, 478 A.2d 755 (N.J. 1984).

[31] Harbeson v Parke-Davis, Inc., 656 P.2d 483 (Wash. 1983).

[32] Azzolino v Dingfelder, 337 S.E.2d 528 (N.C. 1985).

ELSEVIER
SAUNDERS

CLINICS IN
PERINATOLOGY

Clin Perinatol 34 (2007) 299–308

Medical Legal Issues in Obstetric Ultrasound

Frank A. Chervenak, MD[a],*,
Judith L. Chervenak, MD, JD[b,c]

[a]*Department of Obstetrics and Gynecology, Joan and Sanford I. Weill Medical
College of Cornell University, The New York Presbyterian Hospital,
525 East 68th Street, Box 122, New York, NY 10021, USA*
[b]*Heidell, Pittoni, Murphy & Bach, LLP, 99 Park Avenue, New York, NY 10016, USA*
[c]*New York University School of Medicine, 550 First Avenue, New York, NY 10016, USA*

More than any other innovation, ultrasound has revolutionized the practice of obstetrics and gynecology in one generation. Unfortunately, there are medical-legal risks of which all practitioners should be aware.

Obstetric ultrasound plays an important and increasingly frequent role in legal actions, either as the focus in a case alleging wrongful birth, in which an anomaly was not diagnosed and the mother was deprived of a chance to terminate her pregnancy, or as a significant or contributing factor in a case alleging negligent obstetric care with resulting damage to the infant plaintiff or mother.

This article discusses the general aspects of a medical negligence case as they relate to the performance of the obstetric ultrasound examination, summarizes the recommendations of the American College of Obstetrics and Gynecology (ACOG) and the American Institute of Ultrasound in Medicine (AIUM) regarding the performance of these examinations, outlines potential areas of negligence, and discusses ways to avoid them.

Medical negligence

To establish negligence, the plaintiff must show that there was (1) a duty recognized by the law, (2) a breach of that duty in that there was a failure on the part of the physician to meet what was considered to be the standard of

---

* Corresponding author.
E-mail address: fac2001@med.cornell.edu (F.A. Chervenak).

care at the time the treatment was rendered, (3) a causal relationship between the treatment and the resulting injury, and (4) actual loss or damage to the plaintiff [1].

Occasionally, obstetric ultrasound cases include allegations of a failure on the part of the maternal-fetal medicine specialist performing the ultrasound to advise the obstetric patient fully regarding the medical aspects of her case, given his or her specialized training in the field of high-risk obstetrics. The maternal-fetal medicine specialist has a duty to the patient and should define clearly the extent of his or her role in the patient's care (ie, whether he or she is performing only antenatal diagnoses, is rendering consultative services, or is co-managing the patient).

Usually, damages are established easily, leaving either or both the departure from the accepted standards of care and the causal connection between that breech and the damages as the major focus of the litigation. Standard of care is established most commonly by the testimony of an expert witness whose knowledge, training, or experience qualifies him or her to testify as to the standard of care [2]. These experts are limited by the state of medical knowledge and standards of practice at the time of the alleged negligence [2]. Although these standards previously were limited to local standards, standards have expanded to those practiced nationally, given the recent advances in communication and dissemination of medical information.

Although guidelines promulgated by various organizations do not establish the standard of care introduced at trial, the obstetric ultrasound practitioner should be aware of the recommendations of the ACOG and the AIUM. These organizations have published recommendations regarding guidelines, instrumentation and safety, documentation, indications, examination content, and quality control. They periodically issue clinical recommendations. These guidelines are designed to inform the practitioner so that he or she is aware of currently suggested practices in this ever-evolving discipline.

Guidelines

The ACOG's recent publications include a practice bulletin entitled "Ultrasonography in Pregnancy" issued in December 2004 [3] and a committee opinion on guidelines for diagnostic imaging during pregnancy published in September 2004 [4]. In 2003, the AIUM published a practice guideline for the performance of an antepartum obstetric ultrasound examination in conjunction with the ACOG and the American College of Radiology [5]. The AIUM guidelines originally were published in 1985 and now are in their fourth revision.

Instrumentation and safety

Although acknowledging that manufacturers offer machines with three-dimensional capability, the practice bulletin indicates that proof of a clear advantage over two-dimensional imaging has not yet been demonstrated [3]. The ACOG also recommends that practitioners should have a method of storing images and that equipment should be serviced on a regular basis [3].

The US Food and Drug Administration has limited energy exposure from ultrasonography arbitrarily to 94 mW/cm^2 [4]. In the committee opinion on guidelines for diagnostic imaging during pregnancy, the ACOG notes that there have been no reports of documented adverse fetal effects for diagnostic ultrasound procedures, including duplex Doppler imaging [4]. The AIUM concurs and emphasizes the "as low as reasonably achievable" principle; that is, the lowest possible ultrasonic exposure setting should be used to gain the necessary information [5].

Documentation

The AIUM has published a standard for documentation of an ultrasound examination that can be obtained from the AIUM's Website, www.aium.org [6]. These guidelines recommend that a permanent record of both the images and the interpretation of the ultrasound be recorded in a retrievable format and kept in accordance with the relevant local legal and health care facility requirements. They suggest that the documentation include the patient's name and other identifying numbers such as a social security or medical record number, the date of ultrasound examination, and image orientation on the recorded images. In addition, the health care provider's name, type of ultrasound examination, and identity of the sonographer/sonologist should be included on the accompanying report [6].

A preliminary report of the findings may be provided, and a final report should be included in the patient's medical record. In that report, limitations of the examination should be noted, biometric data, including variations from normal size, should be accompanied by measurements, and a final report should be completed and transmitted to the patient's health care provider. Depending on the circumstances, the results may need to be conveyed directly to the patient's referring health care provider, and documentation of this communication is recommended [6].

The ACOG has noted, "Absence of visual image documentation eliminates the possibility of future review or clinical reintegration and weakens the defense against an allegation that an incomplete or inadequate study was performed" [3].

Indications

The AIUM has published indications for first and second obstetric ultrasound examinations, which are listed in Boxes 1 and 2 [5]. When there is no indication, the ACOG has commented that, although it is reasonable to honor a patient's request for an ultrasound, based on the limitations of

---

Box 1. First-trimester ultrasound examination

Indications: A sonographic examination can be of benefit in
   many circumstances in the first trimester of pregnancy,
   including, but not limited to, the following indications:
1. To confirm the presence of an intrauterine pregnancy
2. To evaluate a suspected ectopic pregnancy
3. To define the cause of vaginal bleeding
4. To evaluate pelvic pain
5. To estimate gestational (menstrual[a]) age
6. To diagnose or evaluate multiple gestations
7. To confirm cardiac activity
8. As an adjunct to chorionic villus sampling, embryo transfer,
   and localization and removal of an intrauterine device
9. To evaluate maternal pelvic masses and/or uterine
   abnormalities
10. To evaluate suspected hydatidiform mole

---

[a] For the purpose of this document, the terms "gestational age" and "menstrual age" are considered equivalent.

Adapted from AIUM practice guideline for the performance of an antepartum obstetric ultrasound examination. J Ultrasound Med 2003:22:1116–25.

---

the various studies analyzing the benefits of routine screening and their equivocal results, a physician is not obligated to perform an ultrasound in a low-risk patient without indications [3]. The authors have argued that all pregnant women should be offered a quality second-trimester ultrasound examination in clinical settings where it is available [7]. More recently, it has been argued that pregnant women also should be offered a quality first-trimester ultrasound examination in clinical settings where it is available [8]. Most recently, the ACOG has commended that all pregnant women, regardless of their age, should be offered screening for Down syndrome in a quality manner [9].

Examination content

The AIUM has published a practice guideline for the performance of an antepartum obstetric ultrasound examination in conjunction with the ACOG and the American College of Radiology [5]. The components of a first-trimester ultrasound examination and second- and third-trimester examinations are listed in Boxes 3 and 4 [5].

Box 2. Second- and third-trimester examination

Indications: Sonography can be of benefit in many situations in the second and third trimesters, including, but not limited to, the following circumstances:

1. Estimation of gestational age
2. Evaluation of fetal growth
3. Vaginal bleeding
4. Abdominal/pelvic pain
5. Incompetent cervix
6. Determination of fetal presentation
7. Suspected multiple gestation
8. Adjunct to amniocentesis
9. Significant discrepancy between uterine size and clinical dates
10. Pelvic mass
11. Suspected hydatidiform mole
12. Adjunct to cervical cerclage placement
13. Suspected ectopic pregnancy
14. Suspected fetal death
15. Suspected uterine abnormality
16. Evaluation of fetal well-being
17. Suspected amniotic fluid abnormalities
18. Suspected placental abruption
19. Adjunct to external cephalic version
20. Premature rupture of membranes and/or premature labor
21. Abnormal biochemical markers
22. Follow-up evaluation of a fetal anomaly
23. Follow-up evaluation of placental location for suspected placenta previa
24. History of previous congenital anomaly

In certain clinical circumstances, a more detailed examination of fetal anatomy may be indicated.

Adapted from National Institutes of Health. Diagnostic ultrasound imaging in pregnancy: report of a consensus. NIH Publication 84-667. Washington, DC: US Government Printing Office; 1984 and AIUM practice guideline for the performance of an antepartum obstetric ultrasound examination. J Ultrasound Med 2003;22:1116–25.

The AIUM and the ACOG use the terms "standard," "limited," and "specialized" to describe the types of obstetric ultrasound performed during the second and third trimesters. Standard and limited examinations are

---

Box 3. Contents of first-trimester ultrasound examination

Scanning in the first trimester may be performed either
   transabdominally or transvaginally. If a transabdominal
   examination is not definitive, a transvaginal scan or
   transperineal scan should be performed whenever possible.
The uterus and adnexa should be evaluated for the presence of
   a gestational sac. If a gestational sac is seen, its location should
   be documented. The gestational sac should be evaluated for
   the presence or absence of a yolk sac or embryo, and the
   crown-to-rump length should be recorded, when possible.
Presence or absence of cardiac activity should be reported.
Fetal number should be reported.
Evaluation of the uterus, adnexal structures, and cul-de-sac
   should be performed.

Adapted from AIUM practice guideline for the performance of an antepartum
obstetric ultrasound examination. J Ultrasound Med 2003:22:1116–25.

---

defined by their components, and the components of a specialized examination are determined on a case-by-case basis [3,5].

Standard examinations include an evaluation of fetal presentation, amniotic fluid volume, cardiac activity, placental position, biometry, and an anatomic survey. It also is suggested that examination of the uterus and adnexa be performed if technically feasible [3,5].

Limited examinations are performed for a specific indication such as identification of fetal presentation, evaluation of fetal cardiac activity, or amount of amniotic fluid and are appropriate when a standard examination already has been performed. In such cases an anatomic survey is not necessary.

Specialized examinations include the biophysical profile, fetal Doppler studies, fetal echocardiography, and examinations that are necessary to evaluate a specific question or to evaluate a specific or suspected fetal anomaly or maternal biochemical screening test. Specialized examinations should be performed by operators who have specific experience in the relevant area [3,5].

Quality control

Following the results of the Routine Antenatal Diagnostic Imaging with Ultrasound trial published in 1993 [10] and other studies indicating that the detection of anomalies depends on the experience of the operator, the AIUM began to offer voluntary medical facility accreditation for ultrasound practices. This process reviews the qualifications of facilities'' practitioners, the type of equipment and its maintenance (including the proper methods of

Box 4. Contents of a standard second- and third-trimester obstetric ultrasound examination

Fetal cardiac activity, number, and presentation should be reported.

A qualitative or semiquantitative estimate of amniotic fluid volume should be reported.

The placental location, appearance, and relationship to the internal cervical os should be recorded. The umbilical cord should be imaged, and the number of vessels in the cord should be evaluated when possible.

Gestational age should be assessed.

Fetal weight should be estimated.

Maternal anatomy: the uterus and adnexal structures should be evaluated.

A fetal anatomic survey should be performed. The following areas of assessment represent the essential elements of a standard examination of fetal anatomy. A more detailed fetal anatomic examination may be necessary if an abnormality or suspected abnormality is found on the standard examination.

Head and neck
    Cerebellum
    Choroid plexus
    Cisterna magna
    Lateral cerebral ventricles
    Midline falx
    Midline falx

Chest
    The basic cardiac examination includes a four-chamber view of the fetal heart.
    If technically feasible, an extended basic cardiac examination also can be attempted to evaluate both outflow tracts.

Abdomen
    Stomach (presence, size, and sinus)
    Kidneys
    Bladder
    Umbilical cord insertion site into the fetal abdomen
    Umbilical cord vessel number

Spine
    Cervical, thoracic, lumbar, and sacral spine

Extremities
    Legs and arms (presence or absence)

Gender: Medically indicated in low-risk pregnancies only
for evaluation of multiple gestations

_____

Adapted from AIUM practice guideline for the performance of an antepartum
obstetric ultrasound examination, J Ultrasound Med 2003;22:1116–25.

antimicrobial cleaning and/or chemical sterilization and storing of trans-
ducers to prevent contamination between patients), and methods of report-
ing and storage [11].

The acquisition and maintenance of such accreditation ensures compliance with current organizational standards, is recommended, and often is
required for reimbursement for obstetric ultrasound studies by various insurance companies. A recent study in which practices that sought and received accreditation were re-evaluated 3 years later found that these
practices had improved compliance with accepted standards and concluded
that this improvement would enhance the quality of the practice [11].

Litigation related to ultrasound

Sanders [12] has tracked litigation related to ultrasound. This task was especially difficult because there is no reliable system of tabulating legal cases
that are filed, many cases are dropped following the review of a competent
expert, the majority of cases settle out of court, and not all of those that
do go to court are reported. In 2003, he published his latest series documenting the types of cases he reviewed that were filed between 1997 and 2002 [12].

As would be expected when categorizing suits by specialty, those relating
to obstetric ultrasound were the most common of all suits involving ultrasound examinations, followed by gynecologic examinations. Because damages are based on the life expectancy of the infant plaintiff, suits relating
to obstetric ultrasound can be expected to have large economic damages,
thereby rewarding plaintiff's attorneys with large contingency fees. Sanders
[13] found that missed fetal anomalies now are the most common reason for
litigation, comprising more than half of the cases in his most recent series.
Box 5 documents Sander's tabulation of the possible ways to be sued
when performing ultrasound [13].

Nonmedical use of ultrasonography

The AIUM has published the following "prudent use" statement [14],
which was endorsed by the ACOG.

The AIUM advocates the responsible use of diagnostic ultrasound. The
AIUM strongly discourages the non-medical use of ultrasound for

psychosocial or entertainment purposes. The use of either two-dimensional or three dimensional ultrasound only to view the fetus, obtain a picture of the fetus or determine the fetal gender without a medical indication is inappropriate and contrary to responsible medical practice. Although there are no confirmed biological effects on patients caused by exposures from present diagnostic ultrasound instruments, the possibility exists that such biological effects may be identified in the future. Thus ultrasound should be used in a prudent manner to provide medical benefit to the patient.

This position has been ethically defended [15].

Box 5. Nineteen possible ways to get sued for ultrasound

1. Missing the sonographic finding
2. Misinterpretation of the sonographic finding
3. Failure to compare findings with previous ultrasound
4. Failure to communicate the sonographic report properly to the referring physician or the patient
5. Failure to examine the patient personally or to take a proper history
6. Incorrect sonographic approach for a specific condition
7. Incomplete examination
8. Inadequate quality of films
9. Slip and fall injuries
10. Complications from puncture techniques under ultrasound control
11. Failure to obtain informed consent
12. Complications of ultrasound such as induced vaginal bleeding or abortion
13. Equipment complications (eg, electric shocks)
14. Failure to recommend additional sonographic or radiologic studies or biopsy
15. Failure to order a sonographic examination
16. Inclusion of sonologist in a shotgun suit
17. Loss of films, inadequate filing system, misplacement of films or reports
18. Abuse (sexual, physical, or mental) of patient by sonologist or sonographer
19. Miscellaneous anxiety produced by misdiagnosis, invasion of privacy, or other issues.

From Sanders RC. The effect of the malpractice crisis on obstetrics and gynecologic ultrasound. In: Chervenak FA, Isaacson GC, Campbell S, editors. Ultrasound in obstetrics and gynecology. Boston: Little, Brown and Company; 1993. p. 263–7; with permission.

Summary

Physicians who perform obstetric ultrasound can be expected to be subject to increasing legal risk. Although knowledge of and compliance with the published recommendations and guidelines of the ACOG and the AIUM do not offer complete protection from legal risk, they help the clinician avoid litigation and to defend against it. Failure to comply with such standards has the potential to make any subsequent legal case more difficult to defend.

References

[1] Prosser W, Keeton WP, Dobbs DB, et al. Prosser and Keeton on the law of torts. 5th edition. St. Paul (MN): West Publishing Group; 1984. p. 187.

[2] Moore T, Gaier M. Medical malpractice. N Y Law J 2004;1.

[3] American College of Obstetrics and Gynecology. ACOG practice bulletin, number 58, December 2004, Ultrasonography in pregnancy. Available at: www.acog.org. Accessed May 2, 2007.

[4] American College of Obstetrics and Gynecology. ACOG committee opinion, number 299, guidelines for diagnostic imaging during pregnancy, September 2004. Available at: www. acog.org. Accessed May 2, 2007.

[5] American Institute of Ultrasound in Medicine. AIUM practice guideline for the performance of an antepartum obstetric ultrasound examination. J Ultrasound Med 2003;22: 1116–25.

[6] American standard for documentation of an ultrasound examination. J Ultrasound Med 2002;21:1188–9.

[7] Chervenak FA, McCullough LB, Chervenak JL. Prenatal informed consent for sonogram (PICS): an indication for obstetric ultrasound. Am J Obstet Gynecol 1989;161:857–60.

[8] Chasen S, Skupski DW, McCullough LB, et al. Prenatal consent for sonogram: the time for first trimester nuchal translucency has come. J Ultrasound Med 2001;20:1147–52.

[9] American College of Obstetrics and Gynecology. ACOG practice bulletin #77. Screening for fetal chromosomal abnormalities. Obstet Gynecol 2007.

[10] Ewigman BG, Crane JP, Frigoletto FD, et al. Effect of prenatal ultrasound screening on perinatal outcome. RADIUS Study Group. N Engl J Med 1993;329:821–7.

[11] Abuhamad AZ, Benacerraf B, Woletz P, et al. The accreditation of ultrasound practices-impact on compliance with minimum performance guidelines. J Ultrasound in Med 2004;23: 1023–9.

[12] Sanders RC. Changing patterns of ultrasound-related litigation, a historical survey. J Ultrasound Med 2003;22:1009–15.

[13] Sanders RC. The effect of the malpractice crisis on obstetrics and gynecologic ultrasound. In: Chervenak FA, Isaacson GC, Campbell S, editors. Ultrasound in obstetrics and gynecology. Boston: Little Brown and Company; 1993. p. 263–76.

[14] American College of Obstetrics and Gynecology. ACOG committee opinion, number 297, August 2004, non-medical use of obstetric ultrasonography.

[15] Chervenak FA, McCullough LB. An ethical critique of boutique fetal imaging: a case for the medicalization of fetal imaging. Am J Obstet Gynecol 2005;192(1):31–3.

ELSEVIER
SAUNDERS

CLINICS IN
PERINATOLOGY

Clin Perinatol 34 (2007) 309–318

Medical Legal Issues in the Prevention of Prematurity

David E. Seubert, MD, JD[a],*, William M. Huang, MD[a],
Randi Wasserman-Hoff, MD[b]

[a]*Division of Maternal Fetal Medicine, Department of Obstetrics and Gynecology,
New York University Medical Center, 550 First Avenue, 9N27-BH,
New York, NY 10016, USA*
[b]*Division of Neonatology, Department of Pediatrics, New York University
Medical Center, 550 First Avenue, New York, NY 10016, USA*

Preterm birth remains the leading cause of neonatal morbidity and mortality in the world today. Accordingly, it is of utmost importance to gain as much insight as possible into the causes of preterm birth and attempt to find treatments that can help decrease the incidence of preterm birth. It was estimated that in 2002 approximately 12% of deliveries in the United States were premature [1]. Unfortunately, during the last 10 years the incidence of preterm deliveries in the United States and Europe has remained unchanged or has even increased [1]. The treatment of preterm labor is best described as a "work in progress" for the obstetrician. Many tocolytic medications are used to attempt to stop the progression of preterm labor, but "good and consistent scientific evidence (Level A) shows that there are no clear 'first-line' tocolytic drugs to manage preterm labor and clinical circumstances and physician preferences should dictate treatment" [2]. Tocolytic medications may work for a finite period of time and "prolong pregnancy for 2-7 days, which may allow for administration of steroids to improve fetal lung maturity and the consideration of maternal transport to a tertiary care facility" [2]. Obstetricians practicing in non–tertiary care facilities without an advanced neonatal intensive care unit often are faced with the dilemma of keeping the gravid patient on site for delivery and then transporting the neonate versus transferring the preterm laboring patient before delivery. Both clinical scenarios pose significant risks. In the former, the obstetrician risks delivering a neonate in a hospital setting unable

* Corresponding author.
E-mail address: david.seubert@med.nyu.edu (D.E. Seubert).

doi:10.1016/j.clp.2007.03.008

to provide adequate neonatal care. In the latter, the obstetrician risks an en route delivery of a premature neonate before arrival at the tertiary center.

Traditional methods of treatment for preterm labor, including oral and intravenous hydration along with bed rest, have failed to be proven by scientific evidence as effective therapies. There is limited scientific or inconsistent scientific evidence (level B) to support many routine practices for the treatment of preterm labor such as bed rest, hydration, and pelvic rest [2]. These treatment modalities do not seem to improve the rate of preterm birth and should not be recommended routinely [2]. Additionally, many investigators have attempted to define screening measures to identify pregnant women at risk for preterm labor. There is some evidence to support the use of cervical ultrasound examination and fetal fibronectin testing in certain patients because of the good negative predictive value of these tests [2]. Such negative predictive values may allow the selection of a subset of patients at limited risk for preterm labor who can be managed successfully on an outpatient basis without the need for prolonged hospitalization or tocolytic therapy.

Antenatal corticosteroids are used to stimulate the production of surfactant by the type II pneumocytes in the fetal lung, thereby reducing the surface tension on the alveoli and allowing enhanced gas exchange at a reduced energy expense. Steroids also stabilize the germinal matrix of the periventricular white matter in the fetal brain and may reduce the incidence of advanced intracranial hemorrhages. Limited or inconsistent scientific evidence (level B) recommends that all women at risk of preterm delivery between 24 and 34 weeks of gestation be considered candidates for a single course of corticosteroids [3].

Thus, the obstetric literature confirms that obstetricians are faced with a difficult task: selecting the patient at risk for preterm labor and subsequently providing effective treatment modalities for the prevention of preterm delivery. This task is difficult indeed, given limited scientific evidence that suggests "screening for risk of preterm labor by means other than historic risk factors are [sic] not beneficial in the general obstetric population" [4]. Given this monumental task with limited diagnostic and treatment support, the obstetrician must rely on limited scientific evidence and consult closely with neonatal colleagues to derive a treatment plan with the highest possible benefit for the maternal and neonatal patients.

Team approach

It is essential that patients experiencing preterm labor are approached and managed in a multidisciplinary fashion. The obstetrician and/or the maternal fetal medicine practitioner must work closely with their neonatology colleagues. Obstetricians practicing outside a tertiary care nursery setting must evaluate the patient for potential transfer to the appropriate tertiary care facility. If delivery is imminent, arrangements can be made for the neonatal transport team from the nearest tertiary care facility to evaluate and transport the neonate after birth. The obstetrician practicing in a tertiary care facility should arrange for the neonatologist to visit the patient as soon as reasonably possible. The neonatologist can provide the patient with local and national vital statistics and provide the patient with realistic insight into the rate of survival for the neonate. The neonatologist also can provide the pregnant woman with information on short- and long-term minor and major morbidities that can be expected. The woman can take this information and work with her obstetric team in formulating a plan of treatment that is reasonable and realistic for her gestational age and personal desires. Such a team approach becomes extremely important in treating the preterm labor patient with a fetus at the margin of viability. In 2002, the American Academy of Pediatrics (AAP) Committee on the Fetus and Newborn published updated recommendations formally addressing prenatal consultations for impending deliveries of extremely premature infants [5]. MacDonald [5] suggests, "[O]bstetric and neonatal physicians, primary care physicians, and other appropriate staff should confer to ensure that consistent and accurate information is provided to the parents and that the range of possible outcomes and management options for the mother can then be outlined to the family." McDonald [5] further suggests that, when the fetal prognosis is uncertain, decisions regarding obstetric management must be made by the parents and their physicians and documented in the obstetric records. He further encourages the active participation of parents in discussions regarding delivery, maternal transport, and other management decisions [5]. The obstetric-neonatal physician team must approach the patient in a nonjudgmental fashion and provide objective data about the maternal risks involved in various treatment plans and likely neonatal outcomes at certain gestational ages. McDonald [5] states that "physicians should avoid characterizing managements of uncertain benefit as 'doing everything possible' or 'doing nothing' so as not to place a value on the judgment" of the parent. Bastek and colleagues [6], in a survey of practitioners in New England, expressed concern about whether neonatologists are "performing complete prenatal consultation for infants at the border of viability as described by these AAP Guidelines" [5] and "addressing quality of life values robustly, to explain long term outcomes, and incorporating parental preferences during their conversations" [6]. Bastek's survey revealed that although 58% of neonatologists saw their primary role during the prenatal consultation as providing factual information to parents, only 42% reported asking frequently about parental interpretations of a "good quality of life" [6].

Recently, the AAP along with the American Heart Association published the fifth edition of the Neonatal Resuscitation Program (NRP). The NRP dedicates an entire chapter to ethics and care at the end of life. The NRP recommends no initiation of resuscitation in the delivery room with a confirmed gestational age of less than 23 weeks or a birth weight of less than 400 g. At the limits of viability, exploration of the role of parents and physician seems to suggest that, as uncertainty about survival increases, so should the parental voice, with the caveat that until the infant is born and assessed no plan can be promised. The comfort level for neonatologists lies in understanding that there is no legal or ethical distinction between withholding and withdrawing care. Resuscitation can be started in the delivery room and then withdrawn if the infant does not respond or more evidence accrues that intact survival is questionable [7].

Objective neonatal data

A woman in preterm labor is likely to consider objective neonatal data regarding outcome when making her decision to elect or decline treatment. Neonatologists must provide parents with objective and realistic outcome data for short- and long-term morbidities and potential mortality. Survival rates for infants born from 22 to 25 weeks' gestation increase with each additional week of gestation; however, the incidence of moderate-to-severe neurodevelopmental disability in surviving infants remains high and, most importantly, does not improve over the 23 to 25 weeks of gestation period [5,8,9]. Wood and colleagues [8] evaluated all children born at 25 weeks and less in the United Kingdom and Ireland from March through December 1995 until they reached a median age of 30 months. Marlow and colleagues [10] evaluated these children again when they reached 6 years of age. Wood and colleagues [8] found that 19% had severely delayed development with scores more than three SD below the mean on Bayley Mental and Psychomotor Developmental Indexes, and 11% had scores from two SD to three SD below the mean. Two percent were blind or perceived only light, and 3% had hearing loss that was uncorrectable or required hearing aids. Wood and colleagues [8] concluded that "in this large cohort of extremely preterm infants, disability in the domain of mental and psychomotor development, neuromotor function, or sensory and communication function was present in about half of all survivors at 30 months of corrected age with approximately one quarter meeting the criteria for severe disability." Marlow and colleagues [10] further tested these children at 6 years of age and found that 86% still had moderate-to-severe disability; disabling cerebral palsy was present in 12%.

The costs of prematurity to society are likewise enormous. St. John and colleagues [11] conducted a retrospective review of prospectively collected data on hospital and physicians' costs of infants delivered before 32 weeks' gestation at the University of Alabama at Birmingham. The authors estimated the total initial cost of neonatal care for the entire United States population to be $10.2 billion per year, with $9.4 billion spent on survivors and $0.9 billion spent on nonsurvivors [11]. The authors found that infants born between 24 and 26 weeks' gestation consumed 11.4% of expenditures, and infants born between 27 and 32 weeks' gestation consumed 30.8% of expenditures [11].

Parental autonomy

How much does the obstetric-neonatal-parental team allow for parental autonomy in making obstetric and neonatal decisions? How "at risk" are obstetricians and neonatologist for acts of commission or omission that deviate from parental wishes? The case of *Sidney Miller v. HCA* [12] tests the role of parental autonomy in dictating the immediate resuscitative care of the neonate at the margin of viability. Karla Miller was admitted to a Texas Hospital at 23 weeks' gestation with the diagnosis of preterm labor. The obstetric-neonatal team of physicians and nurses cared for the patient and provided counseling. At the time of admission, an ultrasound revealed an estimated fetal weight of 629 g. "Her obstetrician, Dr. Mark Jacobs, and a neonatologist, Dr. Donald Kelley, informed her and her husband, Mark Miller, that the fetus had little chance of being born alive, and that if it did survive, it would probably suffer severe impairments, including brain hemorrhage, blindness, lung disease, and mental retardation" [13]. The Millers told the physicians that they wanted no heroic measures performed, and the physicians recorded this decision in the medical record [13]. Ultimately, administrative meetings were held, and the Millers were notified by a neonatal nursing administrator that the "hospital had a policy that required the resuscitation of any baby who was born weighing more than 500 g" [13]. Dr. Jacobs stated that the final decision was that what "everyone wanted to do, was not to make the call before the time we actually saw the baby" [13]. Jacobs stated, "We decided to let the neonatologist make the call by looking directly at the baby at birth" [13]. Sidney Miller ultimately was delivered, attended by a neonatologist who was not at the administrative meetings. The neonatologist took aggressive actions to save the life of Sidney. At the time of the initial trial, Sidney was 7 years old; she suffered severe physical and cognitive impairments and was totally dependent on her parents for care. The trial court awarded the Millers $29.4 million for medical expenses and an additional $30 million dollars for interest on these expenses and punitive damages, concluding that both the HCA and hospital were grossly negligent and that the hospital acted with malice [12,14]. Ultimately the Texas Court of Appeals reversed the verdict, and the Millers did not collect any award [12,14]. The Court of Appeals ruled that "if the need for treatment by a child who is not terminally ill is urgent, a court order is unnecessary" [14]. Although the Millers argued that there was time for the hospital to get a court order to intervene on their unborn fetus at the time of birth, the court contends that "the evidence established that Sidney could only be properly evaluated when she was born. Any decision the Millers made before Sidney's birth concerning her treatment at or after her birth would necessarily be based on speculation" [14]. The court noted, "[G]enerally speaking, the custody, care, and nurture of an infant reside in the first instance of the parents" [14]. As such, the parents must act in the "best interest of the child" when consenting or refusing medical treatment. As Annas [13] accurately points out, "[T]he ultimate question the court confronted was whether there was an emergency exception to the general rule that permits physicians to treat neonates without parental consent." The court ultimately looked to an 80-year-old Texas Court of Appeals case [15] involving a child who received a tonsillectomy on the consent of her older sister and ultimately succumbed. The question in 1920 was whether the physician should proceed without the necessary informed consent of the parent in an emergency situation. The court ruled that the physician proceeded without consent and determined that there was time to obtain parental consent before proceeding to the operation [15]. The court found that, unlike the 1920 case, Sidney Miller was evaluated by the neonatologist at birth and was found to have the potential for life by a neonatologist who previously had resuscitated infants similar to Sidney. The court stated, "[W]e hold that a physician, who is confronted with emergent circumstances and provides life-sustaining treatment to a minor child, is not liable for first obtaining consent from the parents." [13,14]. The court did conclude that further decisions after the initial resuscitation rested strictly with the parents, barring any evidence of neglect. Such was the finding of the Messenger Court, which ruled that a father was not criminally negligent when he deliberately disconnected the respirator on his 780-g, 25-week neonate [16,17]. The Messenger Court's decision essentially states that "there comes a point with extremely premature infants, where the risk of mortality or morbidity becomes so significant and the degree of burden and the prospects of benefit so suffused in ambiguity and uncertainty that a decision as to whether to institute or continue medical treatment properly belongs to the parents" [16,17].

What, then, causes a physician to withhold treatment of uncertain benefit? Peerzada and colleagues [18] conducted a survey of Swedish neonatologists and another survey of neonatologists practicing in the northeast region of the United States [19]. Seventy-five percent of Swedish neonatologists indicated that when the benefit of treatment is uncertain, they would resuscitate an extremely preterm infant in the delivery room despite a parental request to withhold treatment [18]. The same survey given to neonatologists in the northeastern United States showed distinctly different results, with only 24% stating that they would resuscitate a preterm infant in the delivery room against parental wishes when the benefit of treatment is uncertain [19]. Both groups of neonatologists indicated that "willingness to withhold treatment of uncertain benefit was associated significantly with beliefs about the importance of quality-of-life considerations in delivery room decision-making" [18,19]. The reason for the differences in neonatology practices may reflect the fact that physicians in Sweden are less likely than physicians in the United States to face litigation for failing to respond to parental wishes.

Does fear of litigation influence physicians' practice patterns?

It is well known that obstetricians frequently are named as defendants in medical malpractice cases. The basic elements of a professional liability case require the plaintiff to prove four elements: duty of care, breach of duty, causation, and damages [20]. The level of evidence needed is set at a "preponderance of the evidence" [20], which is more than likely or greater than 50%. After proving a physician–patient relationship, the plaintiff must prove that the obstetrician breached his or her duty to the patient. In the case of a woman in preterm labor, it may be alleged that the physician failed to recognize, diagnose, and treat preterm labor properly or to administer steroids as an act of omission. Breach of duty must be attested to and confirmed by an expert witness [20]. The American College of Obstetricians and Gynecologists (ACOG) defines the role of an expert witness as one who "helps a lay jury interpret scientific evidence" [20]. The ACOG's key criteria for the expert witness include the following: "holding a current unrestricted license; board certified; have relevant training and clinical experience; clinically active in the relevant specialty in the last 5 years; have relevant continuing medical education courses to the case in question; and be willing to disclose the time spent on the case and the fee obtained" [20]. The ACOG promotes the expert witness who is "truthful, non-judgmental, and is objective and scientific" [20]. It is most important that the expert witness provide testimony that reflects the era in which the malpractice claim was filed. Meadow and colleagues [21] described a situation in which a woman at 28 weeks' gestation delivered a 2-pound infant in the early 1990s. The obstetrician was sued for an act of omission, specifically failing to administer antenatal corticosteroids before delivery. The plaintiff's expert at trial claimed that asministration of corticosteroids was the standard of care at this time, and thus the defendant had created an act of omission [21]. The standard of care is determined by the trier of fact or jury and is placed in terms of the reasonable person, based on the case of *Vaughn v Menlove* [22]. The precedent in this case is whether the defendant "proceeded with such reasonable caution as a prudent man would have exercised under such circumstances" [21]. In *Vaughn v Menlove* [22], the court held that the defendant was negligent for failing to maintain properly a chimney that was in contact with hay, despite multiple warnings. This negligence ultimately led to a property loss on the part of the plaintiff. In medicine, the standard extrapolated to a physician is the reasonably prudent professional standard in that particular profession. The expert witness attests to this standard. Meadow [21] accurately points out that "statistics, not memories" should be used to determine the standard of care at the time of the alleged malpractice. Meadow and colleagues [21] showed that, despite published reports that antenatal corticosteroid use rose from 8% in 1985 to 20% in 1990, 52% in 1995, and 75% in 2000, "expert" opinions from a survey sent to practicing obstetricians grossly overestimated the actual use. Meadow and colleagues [21] concluded that "under no circumstances could an expert accurately claim that administration of antenatal corticosteroids in the early 1990s conform to ordinary care in similar circumstances." The authors proposed a simple yet reasonable idea: "[I]n determining the standard of medical care, the legal system should rely, whenever it can and far more than it now does, on statistical data about doctors' performance rather than the opinion of experts about doctors' performance" [21].

For many years the ACOG has recognized the stresses, personal and professional, imposed on the practicing obstetrician gynecologist. In 1994, the ACOG stated that the college has "long been concerned about the psychological and emotional impact on physicians of medical malpractice litigation, especially because 80% of College Fellows have been sued at least once" [23]. The college noted, "[L]iteral adherence to the advice to 'speak to no one' often strongly recommended by counsel" can "result in extreme isolation" [23].

Are physicians' actions influenced by the threat of a litigious patient? Ballard and colleagues [24] conducted a survey of 1000 neonatologists randomly assigned to receive either a "litigious" or "nonlitigious" set of parents of a neonate in peril. Although approximately 90% of neonatologists respected parental requests to "do everything possible" or to "provide comfort care only," their results "demonstrate that parental litigiousness influenced neonatologists' decisions about how to care for extremely LBW infants, causing some neonatologists to resuscitate infants against their better judgment" [24]. The authors found that "once it became clear that parents were not litigious, neonatologists became more likely to favor nontreatment" [24].

Other authors have suggested merging medical and legal standards to develop a prima facie standard of care for treatment. McMurtrie [25] suggests that by clearly using medical science in the form of evidence-based medicine, a particular standard of care can be developed for a certain condition. Failure to adhere to this standard derived from evidence-based medicine would constitute a prima facie standard of evidence, whereby all the elements of the tort are automatically proven. McMurtrie [25] argues that this measure "will provide legal certainty, appropriate medical practitioner accountability, and ultimately improve patient care and outcomes." In contrast to such a "mathematical" model, Fleishman and colleagues [26] describe the "physician's moral obligations to the pregnant woman, the fetus and the child." Fleishman and colleagues [26] defines two types of conflicts that can result between the patient and physician. The first is "the potential for any adult to choose a course of treatment based on her values and preferences that are considered by the physician not to be in her best interest from a health-related standpoint." A "second type of conflict is between autonomy-based and beneficence-based obligations of the physician to the pregnant woman relating to her potential decision to impact negatively on the health and well-being of her developing fetus and the child it will become if it goes to term." This model accurately reflects the moral and ethical challenges placed on the obstetric-neonatal team, often under emergent conditions. It is likely that the complexities of the physician–maternal–fetal relationship will fail to find solutions in a mathematical model.

The future

Cooperation is essential between the obstetrician, neonatologist, and parents, as is cooperation between the medical and legal worlds. Although the American jurisprudence system is regarded as adversarial, potent beneficial solutions can arise from the courts and ultimately from new legislation. Cooperation between the medical and legal arenas ultimately may contribute to the shifting from a tort claim to an administrative or legislative body of law that will be able to effect change more readily. A recent study by Chauhan and colleagues [27] showed that, on average, members of the Central Association of Obstetrician and Gynecologists had to "practice for 11 years before encountering their first claim and had a settlement every 40 years and a trial every 70 years." This study [27] also showed that 22% of respondents did not have any litigation to date in their careers. These data may help practicing obstetricians and gynecologists place this adversarial system in proper prospective. Ultimately, it may be necessary to develop specialized courts (similar to those in the patent system) to handle complex medical legal issues more adequately. Such forums may avoid imposing unnecessary fear on the part of physicians who then will modify their practices without scientific evidence to avoid being sued.

References

[1] Martin JA, Hamilton BE, Ventura SJ, et al. Births: final data for 2001. Natl Vital Stat Rep 2002;51:1–104.
[2] American College of Obstetricians and Gynecologists. Management of preterm labor. ACOG practice bulletin no. 43. Obstet Gynecol 2003;101:1039–47.
[3] American College of Obstetricians and Gynecologists. Perinatal care at the threshold of viability. ACOG practice bulletin, Clinical management guidelines for obstetrician-gynecologists, no. 38. Washington DC: American College of Obstetricians and Gynecologists; 2002.
[4] American College of Obstetricians and Gynecologists. Assessment of risk factors for preterm birth. ACOG practice bulletin no. 31. Washington DC: American College of Obstetricians and Gynecologists; 2001.
[5] MacDonald H. Prenatal care at the threshold of viability. Pediatrics 2002;110:1024–7.
[6] Bastek TK, Richardson DK, Zupancic JAF, et al. Prenatal consultation practices at the border of viability. Pediatrics 2005;116:407–13.
[7] Kattwinkel John. Ethics and care at the end of life. Textbook of neonatal resuscitation. 5th edition. Elk Grove (IL): American Academy of Pediatrics; 2006.

[8] Wood NS, Marlow N, Costeloe K, et al. Neurologic and developmental disability after extremely preterm birth. N Engl J Med 2000;343:378–84.

[9] Lemons JA, Bauer CR, Oh W. Very low birth weight outcomes of the National Institute of Child Health And Human Development Neonatal Research Network, January 1995 through December 1996. Pediatrics 2000;107(1).

[10] Marlow N, Wolke D, Bracewell MA, et al. Neurologic and developmental disability at six years of age after extremely preterm birth. N Engl J Med 2005;352:9–22.

[11] St. John EB, Nelson KG, Cliver SP, et al. Cost of neonatal care according to gestational age at birth and survival status. Am J Obstet Gynecol 2000;182:170–5.

[12] HCA v Miller 36 S.W.3d 187 (Tex. App. 2000).

[13] Annas GJ. Extremely preterm birth and parental authority to refuse treatment-the case of Sidney Miller. N Engl J Med 2004;351:2118–23.

[14] Miller v HCA, 47 Tex. Sup. J. 12, 118 S.W.3d 758 (2003).

[15] Moss v Rishworth, 222 S.W. 225 (Tex. App. 1920).

[16] Paris JJ, Reardon F. Bad cases make bad law: HCA v. Miller is not a guide for resuscitation of extremely premature newborns. J Perinatol 2001;21:541–4.

[17] Paris JJ. Manslaughter or a legitimate parental decision? The messenger case. J Perinatol 1996;16:60–4.

[18] Peerzada JM, Schollin J, Hakansson S. Delivery room decision making for extremely preterm infants in Sweden. Pediatrics 2006;117:1988–95.

[19] Peerzada JM, Richardson DK, Burns JP. Delivery room decision-making at the threshold of viability. J Pediatr 2004;145:492–8.

[20] American College of Obstetricians and Gynecologists. Professional liability and risk management.An essential guide for obstetrician-gynecologists. Washington DC: American College of Obstetricians and Gynecologists; 2005.

[21] Meadow WL, Bell A, Sustein CR. Statistics, not memories: what was the standard of care for administering antenatal steroids to women in preterm labor between 1985–2000? Obstet Gynecol 2003;102:356–62.

[22] Vaughan v Menlove 3 Bing. N.C. 467, 132 E.R. 490 (C.P.), 1837.

[23] American College of Obstetricians and Gynecologists. ACOG committee opinion. Coping with the stress of malpractice litigation. No. 150. Washington DC: American College of Obstetricians and Gynecologists; 1994.

[24] Ballard DW, Li Y, Evans J, et al. Fear of litigation may increase resuscitation of infants born near the limits of viability. J Pediatr 2002;140:713–8.

[25] McMurtrie L. Setting the legal standard of care for treatment and evidence-based medicine: a case study of antenatal corticosteroids. J Law Med 2006;14:220–7.

[26] Fleishman AR, Chervenak FA, McCullough LB. The physician's moral obligations to the pregnant woman, the fetus and the child. Semin Perinatol 1998;22:184–8.

[27] Chauhan SP, Chauhan VB, Cowan BD. Professional liability claims and Central Association of Obstetricians and Gynecologist members: myth versus reality. Am J Obstet Gynecol 2005;192:1820–8.

ELSEVIER
SAUNDERS

CLINICS IN
PERINATOLOGY

Clin Perinatol 34 (2007) 319–327

Litigation in Multiple Pregnancy and Birth

Isaac Blickstein, MD[a,b,*]

[a]Department of Obstetrics and Gynecology, Kaplan Medical Center, 76100 Rehovot, Israel
[b]Hadassah-Hebrew University School of Medicine, Jerusalem, Israel

Multiple birth rates have increased in most developed countries, with a twice to thrice rate compared with the rate of roughly 1% before the so-called "epidemic" of multiple births [1]. For example, the most recent data from United States births show in 2004 a record high twin birth rate of 32.2 twins per 1,000 total births. The twinning rate has climbed 70% since 1980, and the number of live births in twin deliveries rose to 132,219, which is nearly double the number reported for 1980 [2]. Because twins comprise nearly 95% of multiple births, the overall proportion of multiple births has continued to rise steadily, reaching an all-time high of 33.9 per 1,000 for 2004 [2].

In contrast to the escalating numbers of twin births, the rate of triplet and higher-order multiple births increased in the United States by more than 400% between 1980 and 1998, but since 1999, this increase seems to have reached a plateau [1]. Similar trends in twin births but not in higher-order multiple births have been observed in England and Wales, where a clear decline in high-order multiples was noted [1].

These epidemic figures of multiple births are associated with two related trends: the older maternal age and the abundant use of infertility therapy (eg, ovulation-inducing drugs and assisted reproductive technologies [ARTs]). ART is estimated to account for nearly half of triplets and 1 out every 6 sets of twins. The respective estimations for non-ART procedures are not available. Nevertheless, some European registries suggest that nearly 50% of twins follow an iatrogenic conception.

Several conclusions can be reached from these epidemiologic considerations. First, multiple pregnancy and birth are no more curios of nature;

* Department of Obstetrics and Gynecology, Kaplan Medical Center, 76100 Rehovot, Israel.
    E-mail address: blick@netvision.net.il

therefore, their frequency has a definite and clear impact of the rate of perinatal complications. Second, in many occasions the complication could be traced to the injudicious use of infertility treatment. Finally, not only are many perinatal complications more common among multiples, but also the twinning process provides unique complications that are not encountered among singleton pregnancies and births.

The potential of a medical–legal dispute increases when complications are common. The most vivid example is the association between cerebral palsy (CP) and plurality [3]. The data indicate that the higher the number of fetuses, the greater is the prevalence of CP. Moreover, the increase in CP with plurality bears a clear exponential relationship, emphasizing the effect of high-order multiples on the overall CP rate in a population. In a recent collaborative, population-based study comparing more than one million singletons with about 25,000 twins, Scher and colleagues [4] found that, overall, twins were at an approximately fivefold increased risk of fetal death, a sevenfold increased risk of neonatal death, and a fourfold increased risk of CP compared with singletons.

Many of the potential areas where a medical–legal dispute may arise are expected to be more common in multiples than in singletons and are discussed elsewhere in this issue. This article outlines the situations that are characteristic of a multiple pregnancy and birth.

The reproduction phase

Roughly, one in four in vitro fertilization (IVF) pregnancies leads to the birth of twins compared with 1 in 80 spontaneous conceptions; 1 in 25 pregnancies is a triplet pregnancy, compared with about 1 in 8000 natural pregnancies. This risk can be appreciated from data indicating that among infants weighing less than 1500 g, 10% of singletons were conceived by assisted reproduction, compared with 60% of twins and 90% of triplets [5]. Thus, iatrogenic twin or higher-order multiple pregnancies are a risk for patients undergoing infertility treatment.

Assisted reproduction is frequently the end stage after many childless years and fruitless attempts to conceive. As a result, iatrogenic pregnancies often occur when emotional and psychologic resources are diminished after years of infertility. In such a situation, any pregnancy is usually welcomed, regardless of plurality and the risk in terms of outcomes. Individuals or couples seeking information or treatment should receive complete and full disclosure about factors that influence the conception of multiples, the associated risks, and the available treatment (or the lack thereof) for them. The treatment-specific a priori risks of a multiple pregnancy must be discussed, and if multiple treatments are considered, multiple disclosures should be provided. All disclosures must be in writing and must follow the international standards for providing informed consent.

Ovulation induction and ART treatments differ with regard to the potential risk of a multiple pregnancy. In ovulation induction, multiple ovulations frequently occur, and most protocols are unable to control the number of ovulations. It follows that unless a cycle is aborted when too many ripe follicles are seen by ultrasound, the risk of a multiple pregnancy cannot be avoided.

> In what became known as the Frustaci case (Orange, CA, 1985), Patti Frustaci gave birth to septuplets after gonadotropin ovarian stimulation [6]. Of the septuplets born 12 weeks premature, only three survived, but during early childhood, the surviving infants developed CP and mental retardation. The parent asserted that the fertility clinic and the physician had failed to monitor fertility medication properly and to perform tests that could have anticipated a multiple births before conception, at a point when the decision could have been made not to continue with fertilization. The fertility clinic has agreed to pay as much as $6 million to settle the malpractice lawsuit.

In ART, the number of transferred embryos is in the hands of the practitioner. A high-order multiple pregnancy is rare when two embryos are transferred, and, similarly, a twin gestation is rare with elective single-embryo transfer. The number of transferred embryos in ART varies from country to country and between institutions within the same country. Irrespective of the guidelines adopted by the infertility service, a multiple pregnancy should not be surprising, and the potential need of multifetal pregnancy reduction (MFPR) should not be raised in a post hoc discussion. Once MFPR is considered, the risk versus benefit must be portrayed in an explicit way.

> In a case tried Israel, MFPR was offered to a mother of triplets. After an uneventful reduction to twins, premature rupture of the membranes and preterm delivery occurred at 25 weeks' gestation, leading to severely handicapped twins. The primary claim was against the physician who allegedly did not provide the required information about the risk of high-order multiples before transferring four embryos.

Another aspect of the reproduction phase is the safekeeping of frozen sperm or embryos and the failure of the safe keeper (ie, the IVF clinic) to identify the sperm for fertilization or the embryos to be transferred to the correct parents.

> A mix-up at a Leeds IVF clinic in 2002 resulted in a delivery of twins of different color to an infertile white patient. The blunder could have been at the fertilization stage (using sperm of a different father [ie, heteropaternal pregnancy]) or at the embryo transfer stage (using an embryo from a different couple [ie, heterologous pregnancy]) [7]. DNA fingerprinting confirmed the former possibility. England's senior family judge, Dame Elizabeth Butler-Sloss, ruled that the biological father was also the legal father of the twins; however, Dame Elizabeth suggested that the rights of the nonbiological father could be protected by court adoption order [7].

Diagnosis

Although all multiple pregnancies are at high risk for perinatal complications, the monochorionic subsets are at a much higher risk than their dichorionic counterparts. Several sonographic elements are unique in scanning multiple pregnancies; therefore, the skill and the experience of the sonographer are imperative. It is crucial to establish the number of embryos, to obtain an accurate gestational age, and to determine the placentation (ie, chorionicity and, in monochorionic twins, amnionicity).

At the early stage of pregnancy, this elementary information is used in counseling patients about the perinatal implications of multiples with a specific chorionicity construct. With the availability of sonography, failure to diagnose a twin pregnancy seems to be a serious deviation from the standard practice.

> Recently, a $1.85 million settlement was reached in a case where the presence of a second fetus was diagnosed only during pelvic examination performed by a resident who waited 45 minutes for the placenta to be expelled after birth of the first twin. This child sustained mild left leg spasticity, some cognitive delay, and mild motor disability. The claim was that the radiologist interpreting the prenatal sonogram failed to report findings indicating the presence of a twin gestation [8].

At times, it is difficult to scan multiples, and frequently the accurate number of embryos/fetuses in a higher-order multiple gestation is missed. To avoid this problem, it is advisable that experienced sonographers using appropriate ultrasound machines should scan multiple pregnancies. Once the complexity of such a pregnancy is realized, more advanced diagnostic procedures, such as nuchal translucency measurements, anatomic scans, cervical length, and growth assessments, are considered routine in the follow-up of multiples.

Multiples are known to be associated with many potential clinical problems. At the diagnostic phase, one may group these under four subheadings.

Increased risk of malformations

Multiples, especially the subset of monozygotic twins, have a two- to threefold higher prevalence of structural malformations. An anatomic survey by a specialist is recommended because it is technically possible to miss an anomaly in twins and even more so in higher-order multiples. In contrast, chromosomal malformations are not more prevalent among multiples compared with singletons. The risk of the mother to have one affected child is almost doubled in dizygotic twins; therefore, proper counseling about that risk and the estimation of that risk (by nuchal translucency measurements) should be balanced against the risk of invasive diagnostic procedures (ie, chorionic villus sampling and amniocentesis) [9].

Increased risk of preterm labor and birth

The best prediction of spontaneous preterm birth is by ultrasound measurements of cervical length and funnel width [10]. Although this method is not sensitive enough and despite the fact that effective interventions to prevent preterm labor and birth are not available, significant cervical changes may be used to offer patients early maternal leave and to suggest conducting a more sedentary lifestyle.

Increased risk of maternal complications

Some maternal complications (eg, hypertensive disorders, preterm birth, and complications related to operative delivery) occur more frequently in mothers of multiples. At times, the boundary between the natural history of multiple pregnancy and common complications occurring during any pregnancy is not clearly determined. The following cases demonstrate this effect.

In the first case, a Pennsylvania jury awarded $13.2 million to 10-year-old twin girls who suffered serious brain damage and CP in utero, which allegedly resulted from failure to adequately diagnose and treat a urinary tract infection during pregnancy. The negligence directly resulted in the neurologic damage that both twins suffered. According to the lawsuit, the twin's mother contacted doctors about her temperature of 102°F and her concern of a urinary tract infection during the 26th week of her 1995 pregnancy. After her temperature reached 104°F, the mother was rushed to the emergency room. She was given muscle relaxants to stop contractions. Two days after her initial call to her doctor, the twins were delivered prematurely by Cesarean section. The verdict accepted the experts' view that the untreated urinary tract infection caused serious neurologic damage in both twins and disregarded the inherent much higher prevalence of preterm birth in twins [11].

In a similar case, twin boys were born at 24 weeks' gestation and died due to respiratory distress syndrome within 48 hours of birth. The mother claimed that her doctor failed to detect and treat asymptomatic bacteriuria, to assess her for preterm labor during an office visit, and to provide medical therapy to prevent the preterm birth. The physician argued that premature delivery could not have been prevented. The jury of a US District Court awarded the plaintiff $225,000 [12].

Complications related to monochorionicity

Of special note are rare complications for which the average obstetrician may have little experience in diagnosis and treatment. These complications include the twin-twin transfusion syndrome (TTTS), twin reversed arterial perfusion sequence, and impending or actual fetal death in a monochorionic set.

These difficult cases should be referred to centers with advanced diagnostic and therapeutic competence. The following cases demonstrate this need.

> The mother was 10 weeks pregnant when an ultrasound revealed a twin gestation, but the radiologist did not determine whether the twins were monochorionic [13]. A second ultrasound at 18 weeks' gestation noted discordant fetal growth and amniotic fluid volume. The obstetricians allegedly failed to monitor and treat the evolving TTTS. Single intrauterine fetal demise was found on a third ultrasound performed at 29 weeks. Blood shunted from the surviving twin to the dead fetus via placental anastomoses led to acute hypovolemia, ischemia, and neurologic injury. The case was strongly contested by the defendants, who proposed that there were other possible causes of injury and that treatment options for TTTS were experimental in nature and would not likely have avoided the injury to the plaintiff. After selecting a jury in Delaware County, PA, a $2.3 million settlement was negotiated in 2005 and would be held in trust to meet the future needs of the 5-year-old plaintiff who sustained severe neurologic injuries.

The following case demonstrates that many complications related to TTTS are unexpected:

> A 37-year-old expecting mother of twins who had a history of preterm labor was admitted to a hospital at 31 weeks' gestation [14]. A biophysical profile showed a score of 8/8 for one twin and 6/8 for the other, with absent end-diastolic flow on Doppler study. Before a repeat test on the following day, an emergency delivery was performed due to terminal bradycardia in one twin, but the neonate died as a result of twin-to-twin transfusion syndrome. The cotwin survived with no complications. The mother alleged that a sooner test for fetal well-being could have picked up the twin's condition and would have led to a timely delivery to save him. The doctor contended that proper care was administered. The jury in the Fulton County, GA, State Court returned a defense verdict.

In summary, reducing the legal risk involves the appropriate use of diagnostic tools. Caregivers should explain the limitations of these means to patients. Clear documentation of the potential usefulness and the shortcoming of each diagnostic measure as it applies to the particular case is advisable.

Treatment

Multiple pregnancies are at high risk. They are frequently referred to as "premium" pregnancies, a nonmedical entity, but one that every patient and clinician understands. The potential for loss or handicap, which is high in multiples, may lead to the unfounded belief in the omnipotence of the medical profession to avoid all adverse outcomes. This discrepancy often leads the path to medico-legal dispute.

The advances in perinatal diagnostics were not met by effective treatment for every condition. Even if a treatment exists, it may not result in the expected outcome. This does not suggest that close follow-up of a multiple pregnancy is futile, but rather that the expected outcome for a given expected or unexpected finding should be discussed in realistic terms and disclosed in a clear manner.

Most of the specific complications can be treated only if a timely diagnosis is reached. In practice, the most common problems in multiples are the "banal" complications of preterm labor and growth aberrations.

> A woman who was pregnant with twins was sent for evaluation of premature labor at 35 weeks' gestation because of a nonreactive heart rate pattern of one twin [15]. An ultrasound at 29 weeks reported concordant fetal growth, but numbers within that report differed from the cover letter and suggested discordant fetal growth. The admission notes failed to mention that growth discordance and a nonreactive monitor were a priori present. Labor was induced by rupture of the membranes, and an electrode was placed on the scalp of the presenting twin. Over the next 1.5 hours, late decelerations of the fetal heart rate of twin A were observed, and a scalp blood sampling on that twin revealed severe acidosis. The twins were delivered by emergency Cesarean section, but the asphyxiated twin (twin A) developed hypoxic ischemic encephalopathy and CP. The case settled for $2.9 million via an unknown Massachusetts venue.

Fetal heart rate monitoring of both twins during birth is common practice. Cardiotocographic monitoring in twin pregnancy is sometimes associated with difficulty in obtaining a reliable dual tracing, a difficulty that can give rise to errors linked to double recording of the same heart rate or inadvertent recording of the maternal heart rate that can be erroneously interpreted as fetal. In many cases, the allegation is failure to react to signs of fetal distress.

> A woman at 35.5 weeks' gestation with twins was sent to the hospital because of reduced fetal movements [16]. The admission monitor allegedly showed signs of fetal distress. A Cesarean delivery was performed 6 hours later, and one of the twins developed hypoxic ischemic brain damage. The claim was that the delay in delivery resulted in the injury, whereas the physician argued that damage occurred before admission to the hospital. The jury (Cook County, IL, Circuit Court) returned a defense verdict, and the hospital settled with the plaintiff for a confidential amount.

Another example (Kings County, NY, Supreme Court) is related to the difficulty in assessing the intrapartum condition of both twins.

> Labor was assessed by continuous fetal monitoring for 20 hours before delivery of the first twin [17]. Contractions ceased thereafter, and oxytocin was administered. The second twin was monitored intermittently every 3 to 4 minutes and was noted to have a good fetal heartbeat. At about 42 minutes later, the second infant was born with a relatively low Apgar score and eventually suffered from CP. The mother claimed that the fetal heart rate tracings showed decelerations for 2 hours before delivery of the first

child, which warranted a Cesarean delivery for both twins. In addition, she argued that continuous monitoring (rather than intermittent monitoring) for the second twin could have picked up the distress pattern and would have led to a timely abdominal birth. The obstetrician alleged that adequate care was provided and that intermittent monitoring is as reliable as continuous monitoring. He maintained that there was no distress pattern, and therefore a Cesarean delivery was not indicated. The pediatric neurologist believed that brain damage occurred in utero before the 35th week of gestation. The jury awarded the plaintiff $61,662,500.

The risk of complex intrauterine maneuvers should be anticipated, as the following verdict from a Summit County (Ohio) Common Pleas Court suggests:

> After the delivery of the presenting twin, a breech presentation of the second twin was discovered, and the obstetrician attempted to perform an internal rotation for a vaginal delivery [18]. During the maneuver, the umbilical cord allegedly tightened around the fetal neck. The second twin was born by Cesarean delivery19 minutes later, by which time he became hypoxic and developed CP. The plaintiff's claim was that the delay in Cesarean delivery led to the infant's injuries, whereas the physician maintained that proper care was provided and that the injuries are known risks of breech birth. The jury awarded the plaintiff $3.3 million.

Summary

Liability for the plaintiff's damages is based on departure from good and accepted medical practice and causal relationship between the injury and the alleged negligence of the physician. In the case of multiple pregnancy, some of the issues considered by many clinicians as axiomatic truisms are no more than an educated speculation. For example, inert-twin vascular anastomoses in monochorionic placentas are accepted as a component of the mechanism behind the serious damage to a survivor after fetal death of its cotwin. As recently as the beginning of the 1990s, it was believed that the dead fetus transfuses some ill-defined, thromboplastin-like material to the survivor. Damage was assumed to occur via embolization of vital organs, and this mechanism of injury led to the so-called diagnosis of "twin embolization syndrome." Only in the mid-1990s was it realized that such damage is ischemic in nature and is caused by abrupt shunting of blood from the survivor to the low-resistance circulation of the dead fetus. This new mechanism of injury is imperfect because it is unknown when this shunt occurs. It is as possible that the acute shunt occurs after death as at some unknown time before demise, when the blood pressure drops in the dying or frail fetus. It is also conceivable that a sudden drop in blood pressure occurs in one twin and causes an abrupt shunt and ischemic injury in the other twin even without fetal death. In the latter circumstance, one or both of the live-born twins may be handicapped, and this injury cannot be related to departure from accepted medical practice.

In this article, several examples are discussed in which departure from the standard of care of multiple pregnancies were the basis of the allegation. It seems that the standard of care is not much different from that in singletons, provided that the "high-risk" connotation is acknowledged from the outset. It is not expected that the average clinician, or even the average maternal-fetal medicine specialist, will be trained in dealing with all the complexities of a multiple pregnancy, but failure to perform the basic and standard follow-up often misses the complication and the chance of a timely referral to a center experienced in the diagnosis and management of these complexities of a multiple pregnancy. In many instances, this failure bridges the gap between departure and damages necessary to obtain a verdict.

References

[1] Blickstein I, Keith LG. The decreased rates of triplet births: temporal trends and biologic speculations. Am J Obstet Gynecol 2005;193:327–31.

[2] Martin JA, Hamilton BE, Sutton PD, et al. Births: final data for 2004. Natl Vital Stat Rep 2006;55:1–101.

[3] Blickstein I. Do multiple gestations raise the risk of cerebral palsy? Clin Perinatol 2004;31: 395–408.

[4] Scher AI, Petterson B, Blair E, et al. The risk of mortality or cerebral palsy in twins: a collaborative population-based study. Pediatr Res 2002;52:671–81.

[5] Shinwell ES, Blickstein I, Lusky A, et al. Effect of birth order on neonatal morbidity and mortality among very low birthweight twins: a population based study. Arch Dis Child Fetal Neonatal Ed 2004;89:F145–8.

[6] McDermott A. Septuplets heartache: the Frustaci story. Available at: www.cnn.com/US/ 9711/20/septuplets.frustaci/index.html. Accessed May 2, 2007.

[7] Dyer C. Judge backs adoption of IVF mix-up twins. Available at: http://guardian.co.uk/ uk_news/story/0, 3604, 903677,00.html. Accessed May 2, 2007.

[8] Ob/Gyn management 2007;19:1.

[9] Appelman Z, Furman B. Invasive genetic diagnosis in multiple pregnancies. Obstet Gynecol Clin North Am 2005;32:97–103.

[10] Arabin B, Roos C, Kollen B, et al. Comparison of transvaginal sonography in recumbent and standing maternal positions to predict spontaneous preterm birth in singleton and twin pregnancies. Ultrasound Obstet Gynecol 2006;27:377–86.

[11] Duffy SP. Federal jury awards $13M to twins suffering from in utero damage. Available at: http://www.law.com/jsp/article.jsp?id=1145621808494. Accessed May 2, 2007.

[12] OB/Gyn management 2005;17:3.

[13] $2.3 million settlement in obstetrics/radiology malpractice case. Available at: http:// www.feldmanshepherd.com/articles/numbered/67.htm. Accessed May 2, 2007.

[14] OB/Gyn management 2003;15:11.

[15] OB/Gyn management 2006;18:1.

[16] OB/Gyn management 2004;16:1.

[17] OB/Gyn management 2004;14:11.

[18] Ob/Gyn management 2004;16:9.

ELSEVIER
SAUNDERS

CLINICS IN
PERINATOLOGY

Clin Perinatol 34 (2007) 329–343

Medical Legal Issues in Fetal Monitoring

Barry S. Schifrin, MD[a],*, Wayne R. Cohen, MD[b,c]

[a]*Department of Obstetrics & Gynecology, Kaiser Permanente—Los Angeles Medical Center,
6345 Balboa Blvd., Bldg. II, Suite 245, Encino, CA 91316, USA*
[b]*Department of Obstetrics & Gynecology, Jamaica Hospital and Medical Center,
Jamaica, NY, USA*
[c]*Department of Obstetrics and Gynecology, Weill Medical College of Cornell University,
New York, NY, USA*

Electronic fetal heart rate monitoring (EFM) has been used in clinical practice for over 35 years. In 2002, in the United States it was applied in over 85% of parturients [1]. Despite its widespread use, there is considerable confusion within the specialty regarding the application of EFM and the interpretation of patterns (8), and there remains considerable debate among health care providers, lawyers, and patients about whether it has any value. Its virtues are disparaged in various "evidence-based" articles that suggest that auscultation is comparable to EFM, or that EFM needlessly increases the operative delivery rate, but offers no benefit in prevention of neurologic injury or perinatal mortality [2–6]. A publication from the American College of Obstetricians and Gynecologists affirms no benefit of EFM over intermittent auscultation of the fetal heart, but, paradoxically, recommends its application in certain high-risk pregnancies [1]. It further suggests several temporizing measures in the face of "persistently nonreassuring" patterns, but fails to describe any indication for delivery on the basis of the fetal heart rate (FHR) patterns.

Other articles and editorials have denigrated or summarily dismissed opinions and expert testimony surrounding EFM in obstetric malpractice cases involving babies who have neonatal encephalopathies [2–5,7–9]. It even suggests that reinterpretation of FHR patterns knowing the neonatal outcome is not reliable and even unfair [1]. Such an approach would hamper communications, peer review, quality improvement, and our ability to refine our understanding of EFM.

* Corresponding author. 6345 Balboa Blvd. Bldg II/Suite 245, Encino, CA 91316.
E-mail address: bpminc@aol.com (B.S. Schifrin).

0095-5108/07/$ - see front matter © 2007 Published by Elsevier Inc.
doi:10.1016/j.clp.2007.03.010
perinatology.theclinics.com

Pertinently, these articles and editorials do not call for the abandonment of EFM. That exhortation arrived in a Stanford Law Review article by Lent [10], who argued that the widespread use of EFM is medically and legally unsound, that obstetricians have an obligation to "adopt auscultation as the new standard of care, with no excuses left to defend the continued use of EFM."

Notwithstanding these developments, many lawsuits still involve allegations (and rebuttals) that the obstetrician either failed to recognize or act upon abnormal FHR patterns and that failure resulted in perinatal brain injury that could have been prevented. It was also inevitable that in a medicolegal case, the defense attorneys, assisted by the testimony of board-certified obstetricians, would request a "Frye hearing" in an attempt to exclude the EFM tracing from the trial, claiming the evidence shows that EFM is "junk science" and that the interpretation of patterns is "unscientific." The motion was denied, and the FHR tracing and its interpretation were permitted.

Part of the difficulty for the courts and for the practitioner is that the EFM polemic has not only created some implausible definitions and contradictory positions, but in attempting to compromise expert witnesses and the value of EFM, it has, curiously, also cast doubt on the benefit of care provided by physicians and nurses during labor. It is unfathomable to read an obstetrician's statement that "no proven intrapartum policy (including the use of EFM) can reduce the risk of [neurologic] injury" [11]. In one recent case, the defense expert testified that, as a universal proposition, obstetrical care during labor was "without any benefit". This testimony was ridiculed by the judge.

To understand the benefits and limitations of EFM and its potential role in a malpractice case, it is necessary to review aspects of intrapartum care and EFM (and its pitfalls) in the genesis of fetal neurologic injury and in the pronouncements of expert witnesses in malpractice cases. It is beyond the scope of this article to critique the various aforementioned studies. The interested reader is referred to several articles dealing with their assertions [12–19].

Nomenclature

An obvious problem with EFM is its lack of standardized nomenclature. American College of Obstetricians and Gynecologists properly recommended that the term *fetal distress* be replaced because of its lack of specificity and in part because it is used to the disadvantage of the health care provider in a courtroom [20]. Unfortunately, the now popular term *nonreassuring heart rate pattern* is even less specific. Similarly, *hyperstimulation* has been defined in several ways. In one, hyperstimulation simply refers to excessive uterine activity. In another, excessive uterine activity must be accompanied by an adverse fetal response [21]. Safety would seem to require that excessive uterine activity be curtailed irrespective of its impact on the fetal heart rate. It threatens the fetus with hypoxic and mechanical assaults and does not speed up the labor [22,23]. Ultimately there is no evidence that modifying these and other terms has offered any benefit in communication, in the stature of the specialty, or in protection of physicians in a courtroom.

In part because of lack of a standardized nomenclature, there has been reported a wide range of inter- and intraobserver variation in the interpretation of fetal heart rate patterns, even among experts [1]. This is usually exploited by the defense in medicolegal deliberations. Even the randomized trials of EFM failed to provide any consistent unambiguous definitions of the FHR patterns upon which the evaluations and management were based [24]. In a sense, the randomized controlled trials were premature. They used incompatible nomenclatures and nonreproducible strategies for intervention [25].

To correct this problem, the National Institutes of Health (NIH) Research Planning Workshop proposed a standardized set of definitions [26]. The committee defined a series of isolated cardiotachometric phenomena (decelerations, accelerations, and so forth), which, however important, were proffered without any physiologic or clinical context for the evaluation of heart rate patterns. Under these circumstances, they offer little benefit to the health care provider or the lawyer in the individual case. One might argue that after 35 years of use, tens of millions of tracings, and thousands of articles and experiments, it is too late to make "no assumptions [about] patterns or their relationship to hypoxemia or metabolic acidemia" [26]. Why then use the technique at all or make any effort to standardize it?

The authors resort to EFM as the primary screening test for intrapartum fetal asphyxia because of the limited predictive value of any other clinical risk factors during labor-including auscultation. It is implausible that auscultation and EFM are indeed equivalent [24]. EFM permits continuous accurate monitoring, permits using the fetus as its own control, evaluates tolerance of a fetus to stress of the individual uterine contraction, and permits the diagnosis of potentially catastrophic events in a timely fashion. It limits the application of potentially compromising techniques to the demonstrably normal fetus. There is no example of hypoxia or death on a monitor without warning. It provides a permanent record, subject to later review. With regard to auscultation, there is no study that supports the contention that auscultation is a reliable determinant of the fetal condition or of the need to intervene [27–29]. Even those who find EFM useless for the purpose of preventing injury or death concede its ability to detect fetal hypoxia [30]. Indeed, a quality tracing, properly interpreted, is highly reliable for the accurate prediction of fetal hypoxia [31].

Beyond the issue of nomenclature, there are common pitfalls that affect the use of EFM and compromise the evaluation of its benefits. The first comes when the decision to employ EFM is based on the stratification of patients into "high" and "low" risk. So-called "low-risk" patients account for at least 25% to 50% of newborns suffering from the consequences of intrapartum fetal asphyxia [31,32]. Second, poor quality tracings or unintentional recording of the maternal heart rate, especially during the expulsive stage of labor, reduce the ability to recognize fetal oxygen deprivation. Mistaking the maternal heart rate for the fetal has led to some disastrous outcomes and has become a common allegation in malpractice cases [33,34].

Also compromising the goal of the timely prevention of fetal asphyxia or injury are the notions (and common defense positions) that "fetal monitoring only tells you about hypoxia" and that "it is reasonable to wait to intervene until decelerations are accompanied by decreased variability." Unfortunately, absent baseline fetal heart rate variability is almost uniformly associated with acidosis, cerebral dysfunction, and, in some cases, brain damage [31,35]. Indeed, alterations in baseline rate and increased variability in response to decelerations are often earlier determinants of deterioration than is loss of variability [35,36]. The amount of time needed to prevent fetal injury once variability is lost is unknown. Therefore, if hypoxia and injury are to be prevented, intervention (but not necessarily delivery) should reasonably occur before the disappearance of variability. In some circumstances, waiting until variability disappears may diminish the chances for resuscitation and normal outcome.

But the confident prediction of acidosis, or the prevention of severe asphyxia, cannot be the only goal of EFM, in part because much, if not most, hypoxic–ischemic injury during labor is not associated with profound metabolic acidosis [37–43]. Experimental and clinical observations attest that fetal injury occurs, for example, with repeated cord compression in the absence of significant fetal acidosis or hypoxia [44,45]. Frequent fetal decelerations, as might be encountered in the 2nd stage of labor, especially in association with excessive uterine activity, seem to increase the risk of hypoxia and injury. Moreover, uterine hyperstimulation decreases the options for recovery should the fetus respond adversely. Mechanical injuries may also play a role in fetal neurologic outcome, especially with the fetus in occiput posterior (OP) position [46–49].

Predicting neurologic injury

If one simply classifies a tracing as nonreassuring or abnormal in some way, then the false-positive value in the prediction of subsequent neurologic injury will be prohibitively high [50–52]. Although EFM will not fail to detect fetal hypoxemia, the most fastidious diagnosis of intrapartum oxygen deprivation, including serious derangements in umbilical blood gases or low Apgar scores, will not be a sensitive predictor of injury. Hypoxia is not the same as injury and is a poor surrogate for it.

To use FHR patterns in the diagnosis of neurologic injury [17,18], there must be a basis to believe that the fetus was neurologically intact at the onset of monitoring. Secondly, the diagnosis of injury cannot be applied during a period of fetal hypoxia. As shown by Ikeda and colleagues [53] in an animal model, the prediction of neurologic injury following a profound hypoxic–ischemic event is related not to the lowest pH or even the duration of fetal bradycardia, but to the duration of the brain hypoperfusion (not measurable clinically) and to the FHR pattern after recovery from the ischemic event. Schifrin and Ater [17,18] have defined rigorous criteria for the purpose of identifying the ischemic/asphyxial event, and in certain circumstances, fetal neurologic injury. These data support the notions that a fetus may be injured during labor without being globally asphyxiated; that a fetus may be globally asphyxiated during labor without suffering injury; and that injury may develop so rapidly that it may be impossible to prevent, irrespective of the speed of intervention.

Fetal monitoring works in great measure by helping the obstetrician to confine potentially harmful techniques to the demonstrably normal fetus. As widely acknowledged, monitoring is unerring in defining the normally responsive fetus. Simply put, in the presence of a normal FHR pattern, it is medically implausible that the fetus is undergoing hypoxia or injury at that time. Monitoring deserves credit for reducing intrapartum death, one of the original rationales for its development. But by contributing to a lowered death rate, especially in the premature, it may, in fact, be contributing to the increasing severity and incidence of cerebral palsy [54]. Fetal monitoring may also be increasing the risk of adverse outcome in another way, when the normal tracing in the low-risk patient is allowed to override normal obstetric judgment about the timing of delivery. For example, can the second stage of labor be extended indefinitely with relentless expulsive efforts from the mother but without progress as long as the tracing is normal? It is the authors' belief that the role of the tracing is to keep the fetus out of harm's way, not as the original precept dictated, to affect rescue. The monitor, unfortunately, does not tell you when to intervene!

In many malpractice cases the mother appears in labor with FHR patterns that strongly suggest pre-existing neurologic injury in the fetus [40,41]. Indeed, in a large series of malpractice cases near term, the analysis of FHR patterns confirmed that many, if not half, of cerebral palsy cases coming to lawsuit probably suffered injury before labor [41]. Most of those were injured in the week preceding entrance into labor, frequently in association with oligohydramnios, postdate pregnancy, and the mother's complaint of decreased fetal movement [40]. Such fetuses are unlikely to profit from cesarean section. In some of these cases, the plaintiff prevailed because neither plaintiff nor defense expert recognized the severity of the abnormality in the tracing at the outset of monitoring.

During the first stage of labor, most fetal injury results from catastrophic events such as uterine rupture, abruptio placentae, ruptured vasa previa, and fetal stroke. These problems may not be preventable except by cesarean delivery at or before the onset of labor.

Preventable injuries during the first stage of labor are usually associated with massive uterine hyperstimulation or severe hypotension following epidural anesthesia. Here the pattern may reveal either a persistent loss of baseline variability or the more typical hypoxemic response of prolonged or late decelerations. In the 2nd stage, injury may result from excessive pushing especially with the fetus in the occiput posterior position or in the context of disorders of descent, but sometimes in relation to extraordinary efforts at operative delivery. Here again, the ominous pattern in the fetus may include a terminal tachycardia rather than repetitive decelerations or bradycardia [39]. A significant number of preventable injuries occur during the 2nd stage because, using an external transducer, the maternal heart rate pattern is recorded and mistaken for that of the fetus, whose own heart rate pattern is deteriorating.

There is no unanimity of opinion concerning how to determine the role of intrapartum asphyxia from newborn examination. Because numerous mechanisms of varying acuteness and intensity are involved in the production of injury, and because an individual fetus's response to hypoxia is governed by various external and internal factors, it is unlikely that a single neonatal presentation requiring a critical pH and constellation of clinical findings will confine the timing of injury to the intrapartum period. Indeed, term fetuses may develop cerebral palsy without neonatal encephalopathy [55]. Neuroradiologic studies on perinatal injury fail to support the requirement for severe encephalopathy at the time of birth [56].

These studies further suggest no compelling requirement for severe acidosis or multisystem organ failure to define the timing of injury. The pitfalls of determining the duration and mechanism of asphyxia from the umbilical cord gases have been elegantly discussed by Pomerance and Westgate [57,58]. Indeed, many acidotic and injured fetuses were probably injured before labor. Regional ischemia, as might develop from cord compression or head compression in the second stage, not systemic asphyxia, may prove to be the most common mechanism of fetal injury. Trying to elucidate the mechanism or duration of any fetal asphyxia from the severity of the neonatal depression, neurologic signs or the umbilical blood gases in the absence of FHR patterns is problematic. In the fetus with intrauterine growth restriction (IUGR), intrapartum injury may occur at lesser degress of hypoxia–ischemia than in the normal fetus. Finally, the properly interpreted tracing will not fail to detect any significant hypoxic–ischemic event and will occasionally permit the prediction fetal injury, but FHR patterns cannot define the severity of the neurologic damage.

Despite these understandings, the "essential" criteria for timing fetal neurologic injury espoused in Neonatal Encephalopathy [59,60] frequently appear in the defense in medicolegal cases. This sometimes works to advantage, but the astute plaintiff team will recognize that this defense strategy can be rebutted both on clinical and epidemiologic (statistical) grounds [61].

Electronic fetal heart rate monitoring in the courtroom

In the courtroom, despite the heated emotions that often exist, rational decisions may be made about the timing of injury and the potential benefits of timely intervention and their relationship to the standard of care in the individual case.

The obstetric care provider (physician, nurse, midwife) responsible for fetal surveillance must have certain minimal knowledge about EFM based on the principles elaborated in Box 1. Notice that these principles do not include any discussion about the type of decelerations or such exotica as sinusoidal patterns or "overshoot." If the practitioner has acted in accordance with these principles, it would be difficult to sustain an allegation of negligence, even if there were disagreement about the interpretation of the type of deceleration or the course of action chosen [62].

Malpractice cases rarely depend upon the analysis of the tracing in isolation. Without a proper estimate of the condition of the individual fetus at the outset of monitoring, and using the fetus as its own control in the context of ongoing labor, no proper estimate can be made of the preventability or recoverability of any FHR pattern or any calculation made of the benefit of intervention.

Indeed there are a limited number of conclusions that the expert can reach about the pattern. To wit: The pattern is normal or reassuring (ie, reactive). In this context, the pattern permits the notion of normal fetal behavior and presumably neurologic integrity and absent hypoxia. This pattern cannot be used to rule out macrosomia or malposition in labor, or dictate the timing of delivery for dystocia. Abnormal, or nonreassuring patterns, however defined or implemented, must be dealt with in light of the principles previously elaborated.

At one extreme, the nonreassuring pattern may permit ongoing labor with the expectation of normal outcome. At the other, it may require immediate intervention, either because of the severity of the pattern or because of the improbability of safe vaginal delivery without the pattern worsening. Patterns that may be tolerable in late labor in the anticipation of timely delivery may not be tolerable in early labor or where the likelihood of safe delivery is problematic.

The three patterns in Fig. 1 show prolonged decelerations or persistent bradycardia and would each readily qualify as nonreassuring. The first bradycardia arises de novo in a previously normal fetus, without such inciting factors as hyperstimulation, hypotension, abruption, bleeding, or cord prolapse. There is nothing obvious to correct, and there is no obvious response to conservative manipulations including repositioning the patient and elevation of the presenting part. Immediate intervention is required. Assuming that the infant develops cerebral palsy, how might this scenario play out in trial? There is no obvious negligence in the recognition of fetal distress or the immediate response to the tracing. But if the patient were at term

---

Box 1. Minimal knowledge for intrapartum surveillance

A. Heart rate baseline and variability influence the interpretation. The previously normal fetus will not deteriorate without changes in baseline rate and variability.
B. Prolonged decelerations and those decelerations associated with alterations in baseline rate and variability require attention.
C. Excessive uterine activity and excessive pushing are potentially dangerous. The following limits should not be exceeded irrespective of the response of the fetus:
   1. Frequency, >7 in 15 minutes
   2. Interval between contractions, <2 minutes—peak-to-peak or onset-to-onset
   3. Duration, 90 seconds from onset to return to normal baseline
   4. Baseline tone
      a. Internal device, less than 20 mmHg between contractions
      b. External device, no coupling or other grouping of contractions
   5. Duty cycle[a] ± 50%

D. Monitors have the potential of misrepresenting the rate and variability, and may misrepresent the maternal heart rate as the fetal rate. Differentiation requires concomitant direct monitoring of both.
E. The evaluation of FHR patterns must be made in the context of progress in labor and maternal condition. There must be a plan for the overall conduct of labor that considers:
   1. The health of the mother
   2. The condition of the fetus
   3. The feasibility of safe vaginal delivery.

---

[a] Percent of time (in 10 minutes) that the uterus is contracting.

---

with a neglected arrest of dilatation for over 8 hours or with persistent attempts to induce labor or with an arrest of descent for several hours with extraordinary amounts of oxytocin and the like, then the failure to intervene earlier reasonably represents substandard care. Under these circumstances, it is reasonable to assume that the injury was preventable, not because better interpretation of the strip was required, but because there was no appropriate attention paid to the course of labor and the feasibility of safe vaginal

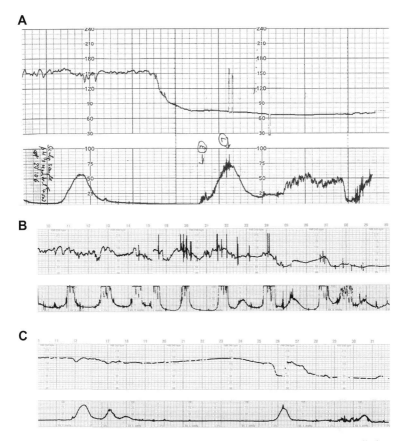

Fig. 1. Prolonged decelerations. (*A*) The prolonged deceleration arising unexpectedly in a previously normal fetus. This was unassociated with any obvious inciting factor such as hyperstimulation, hypotension, abruption, bleeding, cord prolapse, and so forth. Despite repositioning the patient and the cessation of oxytocin, the pattern was unchanged. At the end of the tracing, the mother was transported for emergency cesarean delivery. See discussion in text. (*B*) The tracing preceding this pattern was reactive. In association with frequent contractions and exuberant pushing, the fetus reveals late/variable decelerations that do not return to baseline between contractions. This progresses to a prolonged deceleration with absent variability. (*C*) The prolonged bradycardia develops after a long tracing with persistently absent variability, broad shallow decelerations, and fetal tachycardia. It is reasonable to conclude that this fetus is severely compromised and will likely suffer death or injury.

delivery preceding the event. The timing of the prolonged deceleration in this case was not predictable, but the increased likelihood of it occurring at some time in the prolonged nonprogressive labor was something that could have, and should have, been foreseen.

In Fig. 1B, the prolonged bradycardia develops as a result of the failure to respond to decelerations in the FHR pattern associated with exaggerated pushing with frequent uterine contractions stimulated by oxytocin. Is immediate intervention required, or do the facts of an earlier normal pattern and obvious inciting events permit more discretion in curtailing pushing and diminishing oxytocin in anticipation of recovery? In this circumstance, the authors believe that it would be appropriate to initiate conservative measures—while preparations for cesarean are expedited. Upon arrival in the operating room, assuming that the pattern had returned to its previously normal baseline rate and variability and decelerations are absent, it may then be appropriate to continue with the labor. Irrespective, it was negligent to stimulate the uterus to an excessive frequency of contractions and to permit the patient to push relentlessly in the face of excessive contractions and decelerations to the point of bradycardia. More reasonably, less oxytocin and more restrained pushing should have been recommended with the anticipation of avoiding the bradycardia and the urgent need to rescue the fetus. Experimental studies suggest that increasing the frequency of decelerations dramatically increases the risk of deterioration and fetal injury [63].

In tracing Fig. 1C, the prolonged bradycardia develops after a long tracing with persistently absent variability, broad shallow decelerations, and fetal tachycardia. Does the standard of care require immediate intervention in the expectation of rescuing the fetus, or does the standard of care permit a brief discussion, however compromised by the urgency of the circumstances, that the intervention is likely to be futile and that if the baby survives it is not likely to survive intact? It is not the authors' position here that there is a right answer or that the "standard of care" mandates one course of action. Rather, the authors believe that, with proper analysis and explanation, one could justify any of several mutually exclusive options of care.

Fig. 2 shows baseline tachycardia, absent baseline variability, and late decelerations. The standard of care requires reducing uterine activity, lateral positioning, and supplying oxygen to the mother in an attempt to eliminate the decelerations. Failing this, cesarean section would be indicated. Is the expectation that this fetus will be delivered neurologically intact, or is the fetus already injured and the intervention futile? Would the standard of care be

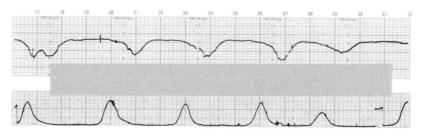

Fig. 2. The tracing illustrates baseline tachycardia, absent baseline variability, and recurrent late decelerations. These features are consistent with an ongoing fetal hypoxia of some duration. It is not possible to determine from the tracing whether or not the infant has suffered neurologic injury.

met by an immediate cesarean section? Unfortunately, the FHR pattern, in isolation, does not answer any of these questions. The answer lies in the interpretation of the tracing on admission to the hospital several hours earlier. Assuming that the initial tracing was reactive with normal variability, stable baseline rate, and absent decelerations, then immediate cesarean section is required in the face of acute fetal hypoxemia in a previously normal fetus. If the preceding tracing were abnormal, the situation would be different. It is within reasonable medical probability that the deterioration of this tracing represented a failure to respond to earlier signs of distress. Any injury, therefore, suffered by the fetus under these circumstances would be attributable to the failure of the standard of care to recognize and intervene on much less threatening patterns, one in which timely intervention would have resulted in a normal outcome.

Assume now that the tracing in Fig. 2 was preceded by a persistently nonreactive pattern with a stable baseline in the normal range, absent variability and absent decelerations. Here the conclusions about the standard of care and the prognosis for the fetus are entirely different. In this setting, one can have no reassurance that the fetus is intact on admission. Under these circumstances, more conservative therapy may be tried and, failing recovery, a cesarean section performed. The expert cannot reasonably opine that the injury was related to the late decelerations, or that more timely intervention after admission would have made an obvious difference in the outcome. At best, the expert may argue that some hypoxia was superimposed on what was likely to have been an earlier insult, the effects of which are not quantifiable or verifiable.

Summary

Despite the persisting debates over its role and benefits, it is likely that EFM will remain a standard part of obstetric care for the foreseeable future. As such, it will also remain a focus of attention in obstetric negligence lawsuits. It must be remembered that in most cases the monitor pattern does not dictate the timing of intervention, but rather is used to keep mother and fetus out of harm's way. In contrast to the studies previously cited showing either no benefit of EFM or no advantage over auscultation, there are studies that show that hospitals who use monitors have improved outcomes on litigation-based studies of individual cases (including Joint Commission on Accreditation of Healthcare Organizations) in which glaring failures of monitoring and communication among providers of obstetric care lead to presumably preventable adverse outcomes [64–73].

There is widespread agreement that improvement in perinatal outcome is possible, that the events of labor can contribute significantly to perinatal hazards, and that reviewing adverse outcomes and making obstetric units more reliable in terms of communication and interpretation of tracings will enhance outcome. That notwithstanding, we do not yet know the totality of injury related to the intrapartum period—irrespective of the mechanism. The estimates of the role of hypoxia vary widely, in great measure due to incompatible definitions and limited follow-up. We have some estimates of the role of obvious trauma due to forceps or vacuum, but there are no reliable estimates of the toll of the other factors, nor are there universally agreed upon techniques for reliably determining the precise timing and mechanism of injury [74]. In this respect, newer developments in pediatric neuroradiology and to some extent a more insightful approach to EFM may indeed help us understand these matters and at the same time improve outcome. It seems that we best protect ourselves in medicolegal matters when we protect the mother and the fetus during labor.

References

[1] ACOG Practice Bulletin #70: intrapartum fetal heart rate monitoring. Obstet Gynecol 2005; 106(6):1453–60.
[2] Hankins GD, MacLennan AH, Speer ME, et al. Obstetric litigation is asphyxiating our maternity services. Obstet Gynecol 2006;107(6):1382–5.
[3] MacLennan A, Nelson KB, Hankins G, et al. Who will deliver our grandchildren? Implications of cerebral palsy litigation. JAMA 2005;294(13):1688–90.
[4] MacLennan A, Robinson J. Cerebral palsy and clinical negligence litigation: a cohort study. BJOG 2004;111(1):92–3.
[5] MacLennan AH. A guest editorial from abroad: medicolegal opinion—time for peer review. Obstet Gynecol Surv 2001;56(3):121–3.
[6] Alfirevic Z, Devane D, Gyte GM. Continuous cardiotocography (CTG) as a form of electronic fetal monitoring (EFM) for fetal assessment during labour. Cochrane Database Syst Rev 2006;3:CD006066.
[7] Scott JR. Expert witnesses: perpetuating a flawed system. Obstet Gynecol 2005;106 (5 Pt 1):902–3.
[8] Cerebral palsy, intrapartum care, and a shot in the foot. Lancet 1989;2(8674):1251–2.
[9] Symonds EM. Fetal monitoring: medical and legal implications for the practitioner. Curr Opin Obstet Gynecol 1994;6(5):430–3.
[10] Lent M. The medical and legal risks of the electronic fetal monitor. Stanford Law Rev 1999; 51(4):807–37.
[11] Clark SL, Hankins GD. Temporal and demographic trends in cerebral palsy—fact and fiction. Am J Obstet Gynecol 2003;188(3):628–33.
[12] Shier D, Tilson JL. The temporal stage fallacy: a novel statistical fallacy in the medical literature. Med Health Care Philos 2006;9(2):243–7.
[13] Paneth N, Bommarito M, Stricker J. Electronic fetal monitoring and later outcome. Clin Invest Med 1993;16(2):159–65.
[14] Paneth N. Cerebral palsy in term infants—birth or before birth? J Pediatr 2001;138(6):791–2.
[15] Paneth N. The causes of cerebral palsy. Recent evidence. Clin Invest Med 1993;16(2):95–102.
[16] Volpe J. Neurology of the newborn. 4th edition. Philadelphia: W.B. Saunders; 2001.
[17] Schifrin BS, Ater S. Fetal hypoxic and ischemic injuries. Curr Opin Obstet Gynecol 2006; 18(2):112–22.
[18] Schifrin BS. The CTG and the timing and mechanism of fetal neurological injuries. Best Pract Res Clin Obstet Gynaecol 2004;18(3):437–56.
[19] Korst LM, Phelan JP, Wang YM, et al. Acute fetal asphyxia and permanent brain injury: a retrospective analysis of current indicators. J Matern Fetal Med 1999;8(3):101–6.

[20] ACOG Committee Opinion. Number 326, December 2005. Inappropriate use of the terms fetal distress and birth asphyxia. Obstet Gynecol 2005;106(6):1469–70.

[21] ACOG technical bulletin. Dystocia and the augmentation of labor. Number 218–December 1995 (replaces no. 137, December 1989, and no. 157, July 1991). American College of Obstetricians and Gynecologists. Int J Gynaecol Obstet 1996;53(1):73–80.

[22] Johnson N, van Oudgaarden E, Montague I, et al. The effect of oxytocin-induced hyperstimulation on fetal oxygen. Br J Obstet Gynaecol 1994;101(9):805–7.

[23] Oppenheimer LW, Bland ES, Dabrowski A, et al. Uterine contraction pattern as a predictor of the mode of delivery. J Perinatol 2002;22(2):149–53.

[24] MacDonald D, Grant A, Sheridan-Pereira M, et al. The Dublin randomized controlled trial of intrapartum fetal heart rate monitoring. Am J Obstet Gynecol 1985;152(5):524–39.

[25] Chalmers I. Continuous fetal heart rate monitoring. J R Soc Med 2001;94(5):258.

[26] Electronic fetal heart rate monitoring: research guidelines for interpretation. The National Institute of Child Health and Human Development Research Planning Workshop. J Obstet Gynecol Neonatal Nurs 1997;26(6):635–40.

[27] Benson RC, Shubeck F, Deutschberger J, et al. Fetal heart rate as a predictor of fetal distress. A report from the collaborative project. Obstet Gynecol 1968;32(2):259–66.

[28] Ellison PH, Foster M, Sheridan-Pereira M, et al. Electronic fetal heart monitoring, auscultation, and neonatal outcome. Am J Obstet Gynecol 1991;164(5 Pt 1):1281–9.

[29] Larson EB, van Belle G, Shy KK, et al. Fetal monitoring and predictions by clinicians: observations during a randomized clinical trial in very low birth weight infants. Obstet Gynecol 1989;74(4):584–9.

[30] Graham EM, Petersen SM, Christo DK, et al. Intrapartum electronic fetal heart rate monitoring and the prevention of perinatal brain injury. Obstet Gynecol 2006;108(3 Pt 1): 656–66.

[31] Low JA. Intrapartum fetal surveillance. Is it worthwhile? Obstet Gynecol Clin North Am 1999;26(4):725–39.

[32] Westgate JA, Gunn AJ, Gunn TR. Antecedents of neonatal encephalopathy with fetal acidaemia at term. Br J Obstet Gynaecol 1999;106(8):774–82.

[33] Murray ML. Maternal or fetal heart rate? Avoiding intrapartum misidentification. J Obstet Gynecol Neonatal Nurs 2004;33(1):93–104.

[34] Schifrin B, et al. Maternal heart rate pattern—a confounding factor in intrapartum fetal surveillance. Prenat Neonatal Med 2001;6:75–82.

[35] Westgate JA, Bennet L, de Haan HH, et al. Fetal heart rate overshoot during repeated umbilical cord occlusion in sheep. Obstet Gynecol 2001;97(3):454–9.

[36] Westgate JA, Bennet L, Gunn AJ. Fetal heart rate variability changes during brief repeated umbilical cord occlusion in near term fetal sheep. Br J Obstet Gynaecol 1999;106(7):664–71.

[37] Phelan JP, Ahn MO, Korst L, et al. Intrapartum fetal asphyxial brain injury with absent multiorgan system dysfunction. J Matern Fetal Med 1998;7(1):19–22.

[38] Phelan JP, Kirkendall C. Permanent brain injury. A retrospective analysis of the international consensus criteria. Obstet Gynecol 2002;99:62S–3S.

[39] Asakura H, Schifrin BS, Myers SA. Intrapartum, atraumatic, non-asphyxial intracranial hemorrhage in a full-term infant. Obstet Gynecol 1994;84(4 Pt 2):680–3.

[40] Schifrin BS, Hamilton-Rubinstein T, Shields JR. Fetal heart rate patterns and the timing of fetal injury. J Perinatol 1994;14(3):174–81.

[41] Shields JR, Schifrin BS. Perinatal antecedents of cerebral palsy. Obstet Gynecol 1988;71 (6 Pt 1):899–905.

[42] Dijxhoorn MJ, Visser GH, Fidler VJ, et al. Apgar score, meconium and acidaemia at birth in relation to neonatal neurological morbidity in term infants. Br J Obstet Gynaecol 1986;93(3): 217–22.

[43] Dijxhoorn MJ, Visser GH, Huisjes, et al. The relation between umbilical pH values and neonatal neurological morbidity in full term appropriate-for-dates infants. Early Hum Dev 1985;11(1):33–42.

[44] Clapp JF, Peress NS, Wesley M, et al. Brain damage after intermittent partial cord occlusion in the chronically instrumented fetal lamb. Am J Obstet Gynecol 1988;159(2):504–9.

[45] De Haan HH, Gunn AJ, Williams CE, et al. Brief repeated umbilical cord occlusions cause sustained cytotoxic cerebral edema and focal infarcts in near-term fetal lambs. Pediatr Res 1997;41(1):96–104.

[46] Ingemarsson E, Ingemarsson I, Solum T, et al. Influence of occiput posterior position on the fetal heart rate pattern. Obstet Gynecol 1980;55(3):301–4.

[47] Sokol RJ. Occiput posterior position and FHR patterns. Obstet Gynecol 1981;57(2):266–7.

[48] Cheng YW, Shaffer BL, Caughey AB. The association between persistent occiput posterior position and neonatal outcomes. Obstet Gynecol 2006;107(4):837–44.

[49] Amiel-Tison C, Sureau C, Shnider SM. Cerebral handicap in full-term neonates related to the mechanical forces of labour. Baillieres Clin Obstet Gynaecol 1988;2(1):145–65.

[50] Spencer JA, Badawi N, Burton P, et al. The intrapartum CTG prior to neonatal encephalopathy at term: a case-control study. Br J Obstet Gynaecol 1997;104(1):25–8.

[51] Nelson KB. What proportion of cerebral palsy is related to birth asphyxia? J Pediatr 1988;112(4):572–4.

[52] Nelson KB, Dambrosia JM, Ting TY, et al. Uncertain value of electronic fetal monitoring in predicting cerebral palsy. N Engl J Med 1996;334(10):613–8.

[53] Ikeda T, Murata Y, Quilligan EJ, et al. Fetal heart rate patterns in postasphyxiated fetal lambs with brain damage. Am J Obstet Gynecol 1998;179(5):1329–37.

[54] Visser GHA, Narayan H. The problem of increasing severe neurological morbidity in newborn infants: where should the focus be? Prenatal and Neonatal Med 1996;1:12–5.

[55] Badawi N, Felix JF, Kurinczuk JJ, et al. Cerebral palsy following term newborn encephalopathy: a population-based study. Dev Med Child Neurol 2005;47(5):293–8.

[56] Cowan F, Rutherford M, Groenendaal F, et al. Origin and timing of brain lesions in term infants with neonatal encephalopathy. Lancet 2003;361(9359):736–42.

[57] Pomerance J. Interpreting umbilical cord blood gases. Pasedena (CA): BNMG; 2004. 132. Available at: http://www.cordgases.com.

[58] Westgate J, Garibaldi JM, Greene KR. Umbilical cord blood gas analysis at delivery: a time for quality data. Br J Obstet Gynaecol 1994;101(12):1054–63.

[59] Hankins GD, Speer M. Defining the pathogenesis and pathophysiology of neonatal encephalopathy and cerebral palsy. Obstet Gynecol 2003;102(3):628–36.

[60] ACOG. Neonatal encephalopathy and cerebral palsy: defining the pathogenesis and pathophysiology. Washington, DC: ACOG; 2003. 94.

[61] Apfel D. Using a differential diagnosis to prove that intrapartum asphyxia is a significant cause of cerebral palsy. Am J Trial Advocacy 2006;30:89–163.

[62] Schitrin BS. Medicolegal ramifications of electronic fetal monitoring during labor. Clin Perinatol 1995;22(4):837–54.

[63] Bennet L, Westgate JA, Liu YC, et al. Fetal acidosis and hypotension during repeated umbilical cord occlusions are associated with enhanced chemoreflex responses in near-term fetal sheep. J Appl Physiol 2005;99(4):1477–82.

[64] Williams RL, Hawes WE. Cesarean section, fetal monitoring, and perinatal mortality in California. Am J Public Health 1979;69(9):864–70.

[65] Greenwood C, Newman S, Impey L, et al. Cerebral palsy and clinical negligence litigation: a cohort study. BJOG 2003;110(1):6–11.

[66] Ransom SB, Studdert DM, Dombrowski MP, et al. Reduced medicolegal risk by compliance with obstetric clinical pathways: a case–control study. Obstet Gynecol 2003;101(4):751–5.

[67] Ennis M, Vincent CA. Obstetric accidents: a review of 64 cases. BMJ 1990;300(6736):1365–7.

[68] Tan KH, Wyldes MP, Settatree R, et al. Confidential regional enquiry into mature stillbirths and neonatal deaths—a multi-disciplinary peer panel perspective of the perinatal care of 238 deaths. Singapore Med J 1999;40(4):251–5.

[69] JCAHO. Sentinel Event Alert Issue # 30. Preventing infant death and injury during delivery 2004. Available at: http://www.jointcommission.org/SentinelEvents/SentinelEventAlert/sea_30.htm. 2004.

[70] Macintosh MC. Continuous fetal heart rate monitoring: is there a conflict between confidential enquiry findings and results of randomized trials? J R Soc Med 2001;94(1):14–6.

[71] West CR, Curr L, Battin MR, et al. Antenatal antecedents of moderate or severe neonatal encephalopathy in term infants—a regional review. Aust N Z J Obstet Gynaecol 2005; 45(3):207–10.

[72] Williams B, Arulkumaran S. Cardiotocography and medicolegal issues. Best Pract Res Clin Obstet Gynaecol 2004;18(3):457–66.

[73] Hankins GD, Clark SM, Munn MB. Cesarean section on request at 39 weeks: impact on shoulder dystocia, fetal trauma, neonatal encephalopathy, and intrauterine fetal demise. Semin Perinatol 2006;30(5):276–87.

[74] Towner D, Castro MA, Eby-Wilkens E, et al. Effect of mode of delivery in nulliparous women on neonatal intracranial injury. N Engl J Med 1999;341(23):1709–14.

ELSEVIER
SAUNDERS

CLINICS IN
PERINATOLOGY

Clin Perinatol 34 (2007) 345–360

Medical Negligence Lawsuits Relating to Labor and Delivery

Wayne R. Cohen, MD[a,b,*], Barry S. Schifrin, MD[c]

[a]Department of Obstetrics & Gynecology, Jamaica Hospital
and Medical Center, Jamaica, NY, USA
[b]Department of Obstetrics and Gynecology, Weill Medical College
of Cornell University, New York, NY, USA
[c]Department of Obstetrics & Gynecology, Kaiser Permanente—Los Angeles Medical Center,
6345 Balboa Blvd., Bldg. II, Suite 245, Encino, CA 91316, USA

Most allegations in obstetric lawsuits against obstetrician-gynecologists relate in some manner to the management of labor and delivery; few solely involve perceived flaws in prenatal or postpartum care. In fact, at least 60% of obstetric medical negligence claims relate to events alleged to have occurred during labor and delivery [1]; these account for more than 80% of the damages awarded in suits against these specialists. Although many of these cases accuse the defendant of not having properly monitored the fetus during labor for signs of oxygen deprivation, there is in most cases an underlying allegation regarding proper decision making about the timing and route of delivery. A perspective on accusations relating to the failure to identify or to act on intrapartum asphyxia has been presented elsewhere in this issue. This article focuses on legal allegations that arise from the conduct of labor and the timing of delivery, independent of those related to fetal monitoring.

Although adverse outcomes from the events of labor and delivery that can be attributed to substandard practice are uncommon, when they do occur, the consequences for the affected mother and child can often be profound and enduring. Most of the preventable complications that lead to litigation arise from violation of a few basic principles of intrapartum care.

It is ironic that during the last three decades, as concerns about the number of lawsuits related to the management of labor and delivery have increased relentlessly, emphasis on teaching the fundamentals of intrapartum obstetrics in training programs has waned, in favor of education in areas involving new electronic or biologic technology (eg, endoscopy, ultrasound, genetics, prenatal diagnosis, and so forth). This relative neglect of

---

* Corresponding author.
 E-mail address: wcohen@jhmc.org (W.R. Cohen).

0095-5108/07/$ - see front matter © 2007 Elsevier Inc. All rights reserved.
doi:10.1016/j.clp.2007.03.011
perinatology.theclinics.com

fundamental obstetric knowledge and practice has had an impact on patient care and the allegations of negligence in the medicolegal arena. That is not to diminish the value of acquiring knowledge and skills based in contemporary biology and technology, because they are important, but they should not be gained at the expense of fundamentals of obstetrics and the building blocks of good clinical judgment. By analogy, a cardiologist who understood the molecular and genetic basis of cardiac ischemia but who had difficulty formulating and carrying out a treatment plan for acute myocardial infarction would be likely to have adverse patient outcomes.

In medicolegal proceedings, the courts expect the defendant obstetricians be familiar with the basic aspects of their specialty. It is indeed distressing in the extreme to hear plaintiff attorneys at trial who have a better grasp of obstetric fundamentals (in the sense of understanding basic terminology and familiarity with relevant medical literature) than the defendant physician. Many defendants are flummoxed by being asked to define, for example, engagement of the fetal head or arrest of dilatation, or to explain the difference between position and presentation, or between engagement and 0 station. Equally telling is the cavalier description of labor as "normal" when the milestones of normal progress have not been met.

The tort system

There are many obstetric malpractice suits that are based on questionable theories of departure from the standard of care or of causation of injuries, and some suits involve frivolous or even ludicrous allegations. This has led many obstetricians to view the plaintiff bar and the tort system as their enemies: the former as venal reprobates and the latter a reliquary of inefficiency and unfairness, both woefully unqualified to pass judgment on the arcane processes of obstetric care. Enormous time, money, and energy have been expended in attempts to reform the tort system, with success in some states and failure in others. Whether the enacted changes (mostly related to capping economic damages for pain and suffering) will have a significant impact on the costs of the system, the number of claims; malpractice premiums; or the level of physician stress, anxiety, and financial risk remains to be seen. These changes have not had any clear impact on perinatal outcome.

It has been argued that the tort system did not create the current malpractice insurance crisis and that we should not, therefore, look to reforms in the tort system to solve the problem [2]. The authors agree. The demon that fuels the core of today's malpractice insurance crisis is poor obstetric practice. Meritless suits, unreasonable allegations, and irrational fears are in many respects the side effects of the disease. Without addressing the core issue of deficient practice, it is unlikely that we ever unburden ourselves of the medicolegal albatross.

The solutions are not complex and involve practicing and documenting good basic obstetrics according to accepted principles. The doyen of medical negligence law and one of the country's most successful malpractice attorneys, Melvin Belli [3], put it succinctly and accurately in 1989: Good care, compassionately delivered and well documented is the key to avoiding suits.

The 100% cesarean solution

A recently conceived solution to the problem of labor-related lawsuits is simply to substitute elective cesarean for trial of labor and vaginal delivery. The rise in cesarean rates in the United States (and most areas of the developed world) to previously unimaginable levels during the last decade [4] has been fueled in part by obstetricians' fear of litigation [5] and the implicit assumption that cesarean will minimize fetal and neonatal risks that would otherwise have accrued during labor and delivery [1].

As part of this rise in cesarean rates, a new term has entered our vocabulary: *patient-demand cesarean*. The notion that women should have the right to a cesarean delivery if they request it has resulted from the confluence of several contemporary trends: a heightened emphasis on patient autonomy in clinical decision making, obstetricians' fears of litigation, the recognition of pelvic floor injury as a contributor to late-life incontinence, and a reduced emphasis on basic obstetric skills in training programs. In this matter, complex medical, ethical, economic, psychologic, and legal issues reside that will require serious discussion and study.

From one perspective, there is much to recommend cesarean on demand. (That term implies it is the patient who is guiding the decision. In fact, patients' perceptions about this issue are strongly influenced by their physician's stance.) It eliminates the risk of fetal birth trauma, intrapartum asphyxia, and pelvic floor injury. It is more convenient for patient and physician, and carries low rates of serious morbidity and mortality, at least for the first pregnancy. Some analysts have concluded that a policy of routine cesarean would be no more expensive to the health care system than is our current mode of practice. This sounds convincing, but a policy of universal cesarean would inevitably lead to more maternal deaths, iatrogenic prematurity, neonatal respiratory morbidity, placenta accreta, and uterine ruptures in subsequent pregnancies. The risk–benefit calculus is complicated and must take into consideration that vaginal delivery is only one of the many factors that contribute to incontinence and prolapse, that many uterine ruptures in a scarred uterus take place before labor, that intrapartum asphyxial and traumatic injury are uncommon and can probably be reduced further, and that most multiparous women do not become incontinent.

At first consideration, this approach has an undeniable appeal. Delivering everyone by cesarean is, however, unlikely to protect obstetricians from lawsuits, just as it is unlikely to improve the health of women in the long run [6]. Even now, women who delivered by cesarean file a disproportionately high number of suits [1]. Moreover, cynics who view the tort system as intrinsically predatory should remember that predators will readily change their diet when one type of prey becomes scarce.

For now, elective (ie, medically unnecessary) cesarean is advocated by some and tolerated by others. If this approach is taken, detailed and well-documented informed consent is the best protection against a lawsuit. Optimally, a separate consent form should be developed for use in institutions and practices that accept this approach to delivery.

Avoiding litigation

There is no magic formula to preclude any and all lawsuits. In many parts of the United States, it is a sad fact that being sued is considered an inevitable element of obstetric practice, regardless of the quality of the practitioner [7]. This notwithstanding, it is also true that most cases sent by plaintiff's attorneys to legitimate experts for analysis are dropped at that stage. Of those that get to trial, at least two thirds are won by the defendant physician, although many are settled on behalf of the plaintiff before that.

The overriding principle in minimizing risks of litigation is to practice good obstetrics; it is not to practice so as to avoid litigation. In other words, obstetricians motivated primarily by the goal of doing good for the patient rather than by the pressure to avoid being sued are least likely to find themselves in litigation.

Dysfunctional labor

The clinical evaluation of labor is essentially a process of serially determining maternal and fetal condition and, at the time of each new evaluation, making a judgment about the likelihood of the labor eventuating in a safe vaginal delivery. In this respect, therefore, the further along in the process of labor we are, the more predictable becomes the feasibility of safe vaginal delivery. When that likelihood of safe normal delivery becomes sufficiently small so that the risks of cesarean section are justifiable, further labor is of no marginal benefit. Dysfunctional labor patterns are important for several reasons: they may presage complications later in labor (eg, appearance of further dysfunctions, the need for cesarean or operative vaginal delivery, or the development of shoulder dystocia), and they may themselves predispose to or cause fetal injury [8–11]. For these reasons, labor abnormalities must be recognized promptly and managed appropriately.

A significant problem plagues our specialty. Our reluctance to adopt a common terminology to describe abnormalities of labor [12] has resulted in similar terms being used to describe different events and different terms applied to similar events. For example, expressions like "failure to progress" or "prolonged second stage" or "cephalopelvic disproportion" defy critical definition or consistent usage. These nondescript terms mire our progress in understanding labor and impede communication and clinical research. Given this nosologic morass, it is not surprising that published guidelines for management are poorly adhered to. The panoply of terms used to describe abnormal labor is a serious problem. From the intellectual perspective, it may simply reflect our relative ignorance about the mechanisms of labor dysfunction; from the legal point of view, it often proves disastrous to the defendant.

In fact, only one organized systematic approach to the diagnosis of labor abnormalities exists: the graphic labor analysis described and evaluated extensively by Friedman [8,9,11]. This approach has been embellished and adapted for use in various centers [13], but the fundamental notion of describing labor according to the relationship between elapsed time and the degree of cervical dilatation and fetal descent has stood the test of time. There have been recent challenges to the use of the Friedman approach, but there is little reason to abandon it. It is the system most widely employed and best studied. It is the lexicon about which there is voluminous literature documenting its value, and, importantly, it is the one best known by attorneys. The defendant obstetrician who enters a deposition or courtroom without understanding how the labor progressed in the disputed case does so at great peril.

The evaluation of labor requires an understanding of factors other than the graph of cervical dilatation and fetal descent. Progress notes should include information about previous deliveries as well as about pelvic architecture, fetal position, molding of the cranial bones, the Müller-Hillis maneuver, and uterine contractility as appropriate. Prior obstetric history (birth weights, gestational ages, difficulty with delivery, and timing of previous cesarean) as well as current estimated fetal weight and station of the presenting part at admission all impact on the feasibility of safe delivery in the current pregnancy and should be commented upon in the record when appropriate.

There is a finite number of acceptable diagnoses for labor that is nonprogressive or progressing abnormally slowly, each with a specific definition (Box 1) and each with a predictable association with the need for operative delivery [8,11,12]. For example, a labor with a protracted active phase of dilatation has overall approximately a 25% likelihood of requiring cesarean for a safe delivery. If there is no clinical evidence of cephalopelvic disproportion and the protraction disorder commenced when epidural anesthesia initiated a T-8 (ie, too high) level of analgesia, cesarean is much less likely to be needed; conversely, if there is considerable molding of the cranial bones, no descent or rotation detected with a Müller-Hillis maneuver, and a malposition, the likelihood of cesarean is much greater. At the other end of the spectrum, when a failure of descent is diagnosed in a patient already receiving uterine stimulation with oxytocin, the probability of safe vaginal delivery is probably less than 10%.

Box 1. Definitions of labor divisions and dysfunctions

Labor curve: a plot of the relationships among cervical dilatation, fetal descent, and time elapsed in labor

Latent phase: the period of labor from the onset of labor until the acceleration in cervical dilatation seen at the onset of active phase

Active phase: the period of labor that follows the latent phase from the acceleration in cervical dilatation until full cervical dilatation

Deceleration phase: the terminal portion of active phase dilatation, when the cervix is approaching the widest diameter of the presenting part; generally this occurs between about 8 cm and full dilatation.

Prolonged latent phase: exceeds 20 hours in nulliparas or 14 hours in multiparas

Protracted active phase: linear dilatation in active phase less than 1.2 cm/hour in nulliparas or less than 1.5 cm/hour in multiparas

Arrest of dilatation: no progress in dilatation for 2 hours in active phase labor

Precipitate dilatation: active phase dilatation greater than 5 cm/hour in nulliparas or greater than 10 cm/hour in multiparas

Prolonged deceleration phase: exceeds 3 hours in nulliparas or 1 hour in multiparas

Failure of descent: no descent from early labor until deceleration phase or onset of second stage

Arrest of descent: no progress in second stage for 1 hour

Protracted descent: descent in second stage less than 1 cm/hour in nulliparas or less than 2 cm/hour in multiparas

Precipitate descent: descent in second stage greater than 5 cm/hour in nulliparas or greater than 10 cm/hour in multiparas

---

Data from Cohen WR, Friedman EA. The assessment of labor. In: Kurjak A, Chervenak FA, editors. Textbook of perinatal medicine. 2nd edition. London: Informa UK; 2006; and Friedman EA. Labor: clinical evaluation and management. 2nd edition. New York: Appleton-Century-Crofts; 1978.

Oxytocin

Many, if not most, legal challenges to the management of labor involve allegations of the misuse of oxytocin. The best defense against such charges is to use the drug judiciously and in accord with institutional policies and procedures. Every obstetric service should have a set of guidelines governing the use of oxytocin. While such protocols may vary from place to place, they should be consistent with those of governing accrediting organizations (such as American College of Obstetricians and Gynecologists) and with the recommendations of the drug manufacturer. To be sure, there is great variation in the perceived indications for use of oxytocin and for its dose schedule among institutions. Any guidelines should (among other things) contain the following items:

- Acceptable indications for augmentation of established labor
- Acceptable indications for induction of labor
- Designation of who may write an order for oxytocin (ie, attending physician, resident, midwife)
- Designation of who is responsible for monitoring the infusion (ie, nurse, midwife, physician)
- Description of how accessible the responsible attending physician should be to the labor unit
- A definition of excessive uterine activity (hyperstimulation/hypercontractility) that does not depend on the fetal heart rate pattern response
- Protocol for increasing the infusion rate
- Conditions in which the infusion should be discontinued
- Conditions in which the physician should be notified
- Description of what infusion pump and other equipment should be used
- Description of how to prepare the solution for infusion and how to calculate the dose in mU/minute
- A mechanism to ensure that informed consent has been obtained and documented
- Requirements for nursing and physician documentation
- Instructions for dealing with a perceived serious adverse reaction to the drug (severe fetal asphyxia, uterine rupture, tetanic contraction, water intoxication)

Remember that, although oxytocin is commonly used for elective induction of labor (ie, for convenience without any compelling medical or social indication), such use is not included in the American College of Obstetricians and Gynecologists guidelines [14] and is contraindicated in the package insert. Off-label use of the drug is, of course, permissible, but such use warrants explanation in the record.

When oxytocin is used for the treatment of arrest of dilatation, almost all patients who respond with subsequent normal progress in dilatation will do so within approximately 3 to 4 hours of instituting the infusion [11]. There is little to be gained in persisting beyond that time unless some special circumstances exist. If so, the explanation should be recorded in the record.

Vaginal birth after cesarean

Attempts at vaginal birth after prior cesarean delivery (VBAC) were championed by women's advocacy groups and by many health care professionals and organizations in the United States during the 1980s and 1990s. The tradition of "once a cesarean, always a cesarean" was challenged vigorously, because the risks of uterine rupture after a prior low segment transverse uterine incision (usually cited as approximately 0.5%–1.0%) were considered low and acceptable. Moreover, most ruptures were not calamitous and were associated with good maternal and neonatal outcome. There were, nevertheless, studies that addressed the potentially catastrophic outcomes of pregnancy with a prior cesarean. Of importance, many of these risks accrue before a trial of labor or during repeat cesarean [15].

The rate of VBAC peaked in the United States in 1996, when 28% of women who had a prior cesarean delivered vaginally, an increase of approximately 33% over the preceding 5 years. Since then, the rate has fallen steadily and was only approximately 9% in 2004 [4].

The reasons for the emerging distaste for VBAC are complex, but, from the perspective of most obstetricians, the change in attitude has been welcomed. The prevailing perception is that VBAC attempts are not generally justified by their associated risks. Of interest is that no dramatically new and damning risk estimates have emerged; there has merely been a rethinking of the known risks and benefits of VBAC, and the medical establishment and the public have opted to eschew it. (How much of public opinion in this regard has been shaped by physicians and their advocacy organizations is unclear).

VBAC is still a reasonable option for women who have had a prior cesarean. It is one of the few areas of medicolegal contention in which informed consent is usually an important factor in a case. It is vital that patients considering a trial of labor are fully informed about the risks that would accrue to them and their fetus. In this regard, guidelines to help identify good candidates (and those who would be unacceptable) for a trial of labor are available and should generally be followed [16]. The authors' paradigm to help select, counsel, and manage candidates is presented in Figs. 1 and 2. Many physicians use a separate consent form for women who have a prior uterine scar. Ideally, such forms clearly enunciate the risks and benefits of VBAC and its alternatives and are signed by the patient during prenatal care. When she arrives in labor or for a scheduled repeat cesarean, the medical record should confirm that the consent has been signed, that the issues have been rediscussed with the patient, and that she has agreed with the proposed course of action. Absent a specific form, the fact that a discussion of risks, benefits, and alternatives with the patient occurred must be documented in the medical record. This should clearly state the date and time of the discussion and the patient's understanding of the issues. In the authors' opinion, for reasons previously stated, the interaction with the patient should also include mandatory periodic updates during the labor by the responsible physician.

It is important to recognize that informed consent in patients who have prior uterine scars should not be confined to describing the risks of a trial of labor and vaginal delivery. It must include as well the risks associated with prior hysterotomy unrelated to labor (eg, placenta accreta, uterine rupture before labor) and the excess risks of cesarean compared with vaginal delivery (eg, hemorrhage, infection, death).

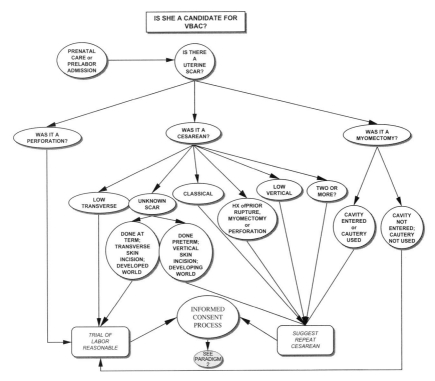

Fig. 1. Algorithm for determining whether a patient who had a hysterotomy is a suitable candidate for a trial of labor.

Documentation

Inadequate documentation is the greatest bugbear in obstetric lawsuits. It is not uncommon for care to have been provided that is appropriate and well within accepted standards, but to have been documented incompletely. The failure to have recorded observations, actions, and interactions with the patient at the time they occurred (or as soon as possible thereafter) permits reinterpretation of the events to the detriment of the obstetrician when the medical record is reviewed later. The interval between the delivery of care and the need to defend it legally may be months or even years, by which time everyone's memory of events is likely to have become imprecise, impairing a coherent defense strategy.

Of particular importance in defending (or preventing) a lawsuit is the quality of the notes written during labor and after delivery. Periodic notes are often absent from the chart, even when the physician has made many visits to the bedside. Whenever a patient is examined, her situation discussed with her, or new plans made, a note should be made in the record.

Notes should include more than just the objective data observations. Progress notes during labor should document what has occurred and

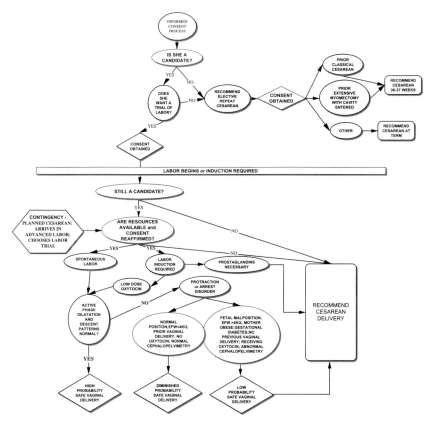

Fig. 2. Algorithm for assessment of the informed consent process and management of labor.

what is planned. They should also interpret what you observed and describe why you chose a particular management route and how it fits into your overall plan (ie, your intentions and expectations). A series of notes should make it clear that the obstetrician has formulated a plan to deal with a situation, and that most reasonable alternatives have been anticipated rather than simply reacting to events.

Consider the following two series of notes for a term multipara in labor who previously delivered a 2800-g term baby without difficulty (Box 2).

The notes from version A accurately describe observations. They are, however, not as complete as they should be and, more importantly, fail to interpret the observations. They do not suggest that a thorough analysis of the situation has been made. In version B, the dysfunctional labor patterns of protracted active phase and arrest of dilatation were identified. Their presence prompted assessment of factors that might explain them. The association of two active phase labor abnormalities, a malposition, and a large estimated fetal weight all supported the conclusion that safe vaginal delivery was unlikely and justified moving to cesarean without a trial of

---

Box 2. Notes for a term multipara in labor

Version A
08:00 Cervix 6 cm.
09:00 Cervix 7 cm. Good labor.
11:00 Still 7. Contractions poor. Start Pit.
14:00 Cervix 8 cm. Contractions strong. Making progress now.
18:00 Fully dilated; to push.

Version B
08:00 Cervix 6 cm, station –2, left occiput posterior. Contractions
    firm, every 3 minutes
    Imp: normal labor progress
    Plan: continue close observation because of malposition
09:00 Cervix 7 cm, station, position unchanged
    Imp: protracted active phase dilatation, probably related to
        position; contractions every 3 minutes, moderate
    Plan: continue observation
11:00 Cervix still 7 cm, station –2, occiput posterior, pelvimetry
    shows average gynecoid features; estimated fetal weight 3900 g
    Imp: arrest of dilatation, malposition
    Plan: in view of protracted active phase, arrest of dilatation,
        malposition, and estimated fetal weight greater than
        previous baby, probability of safe vaginal delivery small.
        Am therefore reluctant to use oxytocin. Have recommended
        cesarean delivery. Patient understands risks, benefits, and
        alternatives to cesarean and agrees to procedure.

---

oxytocin. An adverse outcome for mother and baby from version B would most likely be defensible; one from version A would not. In version B, an expert witness or jury could conclude that the physician did what any reasonably trained obstetrician would be expected to do under the circumstances. He or she used all of the information available to make a reasonable judgment about what should be done (ie, acted within the standard of care). The same, based on the progress notes, could not be said for the physician in version A.

Although good medical record documentation is the key to a successful defense, the content of the documentation is not always obvious. All practicing obstetricians are aware of the importance of this issue which has been emphasized in our educational forums for many years. It is surprising, therefore, that medical records are so frequently incomplete or even contradicting of contemporaneous nursing notes. In fact problems with records are pivotal factors in many plaintiffs' arguments and figure strongly in their success.

It is unclear why inadequate documentation by many physicians remains common, particularly because it so often figures substantially in their legal difficulties. The reason may relate to the fact that expectations on the part of the courts as well as the specialty have advanced. The traditional SOAP (Subjective, Objective, Assessment, Plan) format is most useful in this regard and should be used whenever possible. It is crucial that the physician's progress notes address the following:

1. A description and assessment of the patient's symptoms and subjective feelings
2. A description of the pertinent physical findings, laboratory results, or other new findings
3. An assessment or differential diagnosis
4. A rational plan based on the above

Brachial plexus injury

One of the most common sources of obstetric malpractice litigation is that of newborn brachial plexus palsy. This entity is reviewed here from the perspective of how management and documentation of the events of labor influence risk.

Medical and legal attitudes regarding shoulder dystocia are evolving. It had been thought that newborn brachial plexus palsy resulted from excessive traction applied by the obstetrician and was clear proof of medical negligence. More recent evidence has established that some cases occur in the absence of any difficulties at the time of delivery. As a consequence of this new attitude, the focus of litigation has shifted from the assumption that the mere presence of a palsy is evidence of negligence to the notion that either the provocation should have been predicted based on pre-existing risk factors (and the baby therefore delivered by cesarean) or that the maneuvers used to overcome shoulder dystocia at the time of delivery were employed inappropriately or negligently.

The allegation in these cases is often that the obstetrician failed to identify factors shown in various studies to be associated with increased odds of shoulder dystocia or brachial plexus injury [17–19]. However, most such studies, even those that use multiple logistic regression to correct for confounding, are explanatory models. As such, they are useful to understand what factors are associated with an outcome, but cannot be used to predict the risk of complications in an individual case [20]. This distinction is not used to sufficient advantage in the defense of brachial plexus injury cases.

The allegation that the obstetrician failed to recognize abnormal labor patterns that predispose to shoulder dystocia and nerve plexus injury is also common. In this regard, many have taken the position that brachial plexus injuries are simply an unpreventable and unpredictable complication [21].

In fact, as many as three fourths of brachial plexus injuries are preceded by abnormal labor [19]. Those labor abnormalities most commonly associated with difficult shoulder delivery are characterized by either recalcitrant dilatation and descent or (seemingly paradoxically) by exceptionally rapid descent. Some evidence suggests that certain features of labor (prolonged deceleration phase and long second stage) are independently associated with brachial plexus injuries [19,22,23]. When coupled with information about maternal body mass, estimated fetal weight, and other factors, a reasonable estimate of the likelihood of brachial plexus injuries can be made in advance of delivery [24].

There is no doubt that almost all cases of shoulder dystocia and its attendant serious complications could be avoided by performing cesarean delivery. The pertinent question is thus not whether shoulder dystocia can be prevented, but rather how much serious injury will occur when it is ideally managed. It then becomes relevant to ask how many unnecessary cesarean deliveries would be required to prevent each case. Optimal means to address that question are not yet available, but may evolve as logistic regression models derived from extensive clinical experience are built from large data sets. Some predictive models exist but have been tested in limited samples thus far [24–26].

Medical record

Appropriate documentation of the events associated with shoulder dystocia in the medical record is vital. Such documentation allows detailed and accurate interpretation of the delivery by those evaluating it in retrospect, an issue of obvious importance in risk management.

The medical record, beginning with the admission note, should scrupulously record any demographic, obstetric, prenatal, or intrapartum factors that increase the risk of shoulder dystocia. The record should indicate that, when appropriate, the likely risk of shoulder dystocia was assessed, thoughtful preparation for it at delivery was made, and a discussion about these risks with the mother occurred.

From the legal perspective, the failure to identify risk factors for shoulder dystocia most commonly resides in one or more of the following areas:

- Failure to identify risk factors in the patient's previous obstetric history (prior large babies, shoulder dystocia, gestational diabetes mellitus, instrumental delivery, dysfunctional labor)
- Failure to identify prenatal risk factors (mild glucose intolerance, obesity, excessive weight gain, large estimated fetal weight, adverse pelvic architecture)
- Failure to recognize the presence of intrapartum risk factors (development of dysfunctional labor, especially long deceleration phase and long second stage; anatomic features of the pelvis that predispose; large fetal weight)

- Unfamiliarity with the proper way to perform maneuvers to relieve the shoulder impaction
- Failure to document properly all of the events of the labor and delivery

The plaintiff may claim that the physician failed to offer elective cesarean delivery before labor in patients who have multiple risk factors. Allegations that, during labor, the obstetrician failed to recognize abnormal labor patterns that predispose to shoulder dystocia and nerve plexus injury or that the decision to perform operative vaginal delivery was inappropriate are common. Finally, mismanagement of shoulder dystocia when it occurs is often charged. This failure may include the use of inappropriate maneuvers to remove the impacted shoulder, the failure to use accepted maneuvers in these efforts, or the failure to have appropriately trained and experienced personnel at the time of delivery. In fact the greater the traction injury (avulsion of nerve roots for example), the more compelling will be the argument that excessive traction in the wrong direction was used.

The best defense against these potential allegations is to have provided and documented good antepartum and intrapartum care that included the patient's participation in decision making, to have exercised reasonable care in anticipating shoulder dystocia, and to have taken all reasonable measures to manage it if it occurred.

It should be emphasized that if, after discussing the situation with a patient, she desires cesarean section, that wish must either be granted or an agreement to pursue a trial of labor must be renegotiated. The physician may not unilaterally decide the benefits to the patient because, in the final analysis, informed consent is obtained from the patient, not given to her.

Coping

Errors in the management of labor, as in all human endeavors, are inevitable. We make decisions about complex situations and have sometimes to act in situations of greater or lesser medical certainty when insufficient information is available. The vagaries of an individual patient's responses are difficult to predict. Moreover the consequences of medical decisions are often influenced by system problems over which the practitioner has little control.

No one wants to make a mistake, most assuredly not one that could harm a patient. The problem is that we live in an era of finger pointing and recrimination. So, we need not only to learn to avoid errors but how to cope with them when they inevitably occur. Arguably, the whole of medical training and education is geared to help us do no harm. Mostly, we do that well, but sometimes we stumble. How we, as individuals, and how the system in which we labor deal with that misstep so that it becomes an object lesson and a nidus for improvement is key. Ignoring mistakes, or blaming them on the system or on others is not curative. Processing our mistakes so that some ultimate good comes from them requires dealing with our guilt, accepting our fallibility, and using them constructively. Our aspiration to perfection in medical practice will never be realized, but that reality should never dampen our efforts to attain it. The best of us will keep trying.

Summary recommendations to avoid litigation related to labor and delivery

1. Maintain detailed and clear communications with the patient, especially when complications arise. Many lawsuits arise from the patient's need to find out what happened; others are out of anger at a perceived "cover-up" on the part of her providers.
2. Use the Friedman labor curves and standardized terminology for all labors. (If you do not make such a curve during the labor, you must make it to defend your lawsuit).
3. Identify dysfunctional labor patterns promptly and apply appropriate evaluation and therapy, and maintain communication with the parent(s).
4. Follow institutional guidelines for administration of oxytocin, especially in avoiding hyperstimulation or prolonged use.
5. Do not use cervical ripening agents in patients already having regular uterine contractions.
6. Avoid excessive uterine activity irrespective of the fetal heart rate pattern response. It limits oxygen availability, increases mechanical stresses on the fetal head, changes cerebral vascular dynamics, and does not make cervical dilatation occur any faster.
7. Be present when your patient is in labor, especially when there are significant risk factors or complications. Telephone management of labor is fraught with hazard.
8. When unsure, consult a more knowledgeable or experienced person.
9. When a nurse or resident asks you to come to the labor unit, do so without hesitation.
10. Document every patient encounter, including a description of your intentions and expectations.
11. When an intervention is planned (oxytocin, forceps, cesarean, epidural, and so forth), document the informed consent discussion clearly.

References

[1] American College of Obstetricians and Gynecologists. Professional liability and risk management: an essential guide for obstetrician –gynecologists. Washington, DC: ACOG; 2005.
[2] Baker T. The medical malpractice myth. Chicago: University of Chicago Press; 2005.
[3] Belli M. Belli for your malpractice defense. 2nd edition. Oradell (NJ): Medical Economics Books; 1989.
[4] National Center for Health Statistics. Births: preliminary data for 2005. Available at: http://www.cdc.gov/nchs/products/pubs/pubd/hestats/prelimbirths05.

[5] Dubay L, Kaestner R, Waidmann T. The impact of malpractice fears on cesarean section rates. J Health Econ 1999;18:491–522.

[6] Kolas T, Saugstad OD, Daltveit AK, et al. Planned cesarean versus planned vaginal delivery at term: comparison of newborn and infant outcomes. Am J Obstet Gynecol 2006;195: 1538–43.

[7] American College of Obstetricians and Gynecologists 2006 Survey on Professional Liability. Available at: http://www.acog.org.

[8] Cohen WR, Friedman EA. The assessment of labor. In: Kurjak A, Chervenak FA, editors. Textbook of perinatal medicine. 2nd edition. London: Informa UK; 2006. p. 1821–30.

[9] Friedman EA. Effects of labor and delivery on the fetus. In: Kurjak A, Chervenak FA, editors. Textbook of perinatal medicine. 2nd edition. London: Informa UK; 2006. p. 1989–97.

[10] Towner D, Castro MA, Eby-Wilkens BS, et al. Effect of mode of delivery in nulliparous women on neonatal intracranial injury. N Engl J Med 1999;341:1709–14.

[11] Friedman EA. Labor: clinical evaluation and management. 2nd edition. New York: Appleton-Century-Crofts; 1978.

[12] Schifrin BS, Cohen WR. Labor's dysfunctional lexicon. Obstet Gynecol 1989;74:121–4.

[13] Cohen WR. Controversies in the assessment of labor. Prog Obstet Gynecol 2006;17:231–44.

[14] ACOG Practice Bulletin Number 10. Induction of labor. American College of Obstetricians and Gynecologists, Washington DC, November 1999.

[15] Chazotte C, Cohen WR. Catastrophic complications of previous cesarean section. Am J Obstet Gynecol 1990;163:738–42.

[16] ACOG Practice Bulletin Number 54. Vaginal birth after previous cesarean delivery. American College of Obstetricians and Gynecologists, Washington, DC, July 2004.

[17] Mehta SH, Blackwell SC, Bujold E, et al. What factors are associated with neonatal injury following shoulder dystocia? J Perinatol 2006;26:85–8.

[18] Nocon JJ, McKenzie DK, Thomas LJ, et al. Shoulder dystocia: an analysis of risks and obstetric maneuvers. Am J Obstet Gynecol 1993;168:1732–9.

[19] Weizsaecker K, Deaver JE, Cohen WR. Labour characteristics and neonatal Erb's palsy. BJOG, in press.

[20] Ware JH. The limitations of risk factors as prognostic tools. N Engl J Med 2006;355:2615–7.

[21] Gherman RB, Chauhan S, Ouzounian JG, et al. Shoulder dystocia: the unpreventable obstetric emergency with empiric management guidelines. Am J Obstet Gynecol 2006;195: 657–72.

[22] Gross TL, Sokol RJ, Williams T, et al. Shoulder dystocia: a fetal-physician risk. Am J Obstet Gynecol 1987;156:1408–18.

[23] Hopwood HG. Shoulder dystocia: fifteen years' experience in a community hospital. Am J Obstet Gynecol 1982;144:162–6.

[24] Deaver JE, Cohen WR. Test characteristics of a neonatal brachial plexus injury prevention score. Reproductive Sciences 2007;14:241A.

[25] Dyachenko A, Ciampi A, Fahey J, et al. Prediction of risk for shoulder dystocia with neonatal injury. Am J Obstet Gynecol 2006;195:1544–9.

[26] Belfort MA, Dildy GA, Saade GR, et al. Prediction of shoulder dystocia using multivariate analysis. Am J Perinatol 2007;25:5–10.

ELSEVIER
SAUNDERS

CLINICS IN
PERINATOLOGY

Clin Perinatol 34 (2007) 361–364

Index

Note: Page numbers of article titles are in **boldface** type.

0095-5108/07/$ - see front matter © 2007 Elsevier Inc. All rights reserved.
doi:10.1016/S0095-5108(07)00049-8
perinatology.theclinics.com

Moving?

Make sure your subscription moves with you!

To notify us of your new address, find your **Clinics Account Number** (located on your mailing label above your name), and contact customer service at:

E-mail: elspcs@elsevier.com

800-654-2452 (subscribers in the U.S. & Canada)
407-345-4000 (subscribers outside of the U.S. & Canada)

Fax number: 407-363-9661

Elsevier Periodicals Customer Service
6277 Sea Harbor Drive
Orlando, FL 32887-4800

*To ensure uninterrupted delivery of your subscription, please notify us at least 4 weeks in advance of move.